Compact Clinica

MECHANICAL
VENTILATION

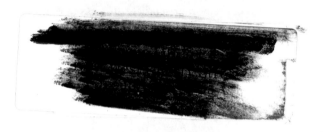

Sandra Goldsworthy, RN, MSc, PhD(c), CNCC(C), CMSN(C), is a recognized leader in critical care nursing and has worked in this field for more than 25 years. She is currently a nursing professor in the Georgian College/York University BScN program and critical care program, and is also an accomplished practitioner, consultant, researcher, and author. She received her bachelor of science in nursing at Lakehead University and her master of science in nursing from Queen's University. She is currently pursuing her PhD in nursing at the University of British Columbia. She holds a national CNA credential in critical care as well as in medical surgical nursing. Her research focus is retention of critical care nurses. Dr. Goldsworthy has conducted and published research involving the use of simulation and personal digital assistants (PDAs) in nursing education. She is currently involved in the delivery of critical care simulation and the mentoring of other educators in this technology. Her recent publications and national and international presentations have concentrated on critical care, simulation, and technology in nursing. She also sits on a number of national and international nursing committees, including the national exam committee for the Canadian Nurse's Association Medical/Surgical Nursing Certification exam. She has edited or authored five textbooks including all three editions of the *Medical Surgical Nursing in Canada* textbook, *Simulation Simplified: A Practical Guide for Nurse Educators,* and *Simulation Simplified: Student Lab Manual for Critical Care Nursing.*

Leslie Graham, RN, MN, CNCC(C), CHSE, is a faculty member in the Collaborative Nursing Program at Durham College–University of Ontario, Institute of Technology. With over 25 years of critical care experience, the majority spent in direct care, she is well acquainted with the challenges and rewards of critical care nursing. As a critical care educator she seeks to translate evidence-informed practices at the bedside. As an award-winning author, Ms. Graham has published resources that assist both the educator and the critical care student. She has presented nationally and internationally on critical care topics ranging from education of critical care nurses to practical application at the bedside.

THE COMPACT CLINICAL GUIDE *SERIES*

Compact Clinical Guide to
MECHANICAL VENTILATION
Foundations of Practice for Critical Care Nurses
Sandra Goldsworthy, RN, MSc, PhD(c), CNCC(C), CMSN(C)
Leslie Graham, RN, MN, CNCC(C), CHSE

Upcoming Titles

Compact Clinical Guide to
ARRHYTHMIA AND 12-LEAD EKG INTERPRETATION
Foundations of Practice for Critical Care Nurses
Sandra Goldsworthy, RN, MSc, PhD(c), CNCC(C), CMSN(C)
Leslie Graham, RN, MN, CNCC(C), CHSE

Compact Clinical Guide to
HEMODYNAMIC MONITORING
Foundations of Practice for Critical Care Nurses
Sandra Goldsworthy, RN, MSc, PhD(c), CNCC(C), CMSN(C)
Leslie Graham, RN, MN, CNCC(C), CHSE

Compact Clinical Guide to

MECHANICAL VENTILATION

Foundations of Practice for Critical Care Nurses

Sandra Goldsworthy, RN, MSc, PhD(c), CNCC(C), CMSN(C)

Leslie Graham, RN, MN, CNCC(C), CHSE

SPRINGER PUBLISHING COMPANY
NEW YORK

Springer Publishing Company, LLC
11 West 42nd Street
New York, NY 10036
www.springerpub.com

Acquisitions Editor: Elizabeth Nieginski
Composition: S4Carlisle

ISBN: 978-0-8261-9806-8
e-book ISBN: 978-0-8261-9807-5

13 14 15 16 17 / 5 4 3 2 1

The author and the publisher of this Work have made every effort to use sources believed to be reliable to provide information that is accurate and compatible with the standards generally accepted at the time of publication. Because medical science is continually advancing, our knowledge base continues to expand. Therefore, as new information becomes available, changes in procedures become necessary. We recommend that the reader always consult current research and specific institutional policies before performing any clinical procedure. The author and publisher shall not be liable for any special, consequential, or exemplary damages resulting, in whole or in part, from the readers' use of, or reliance on, the information contained in this book. The publisher has no responsibility for the persistence or accuracy of URLs for external or third-party Internet websites referred to in this publication and does not guarantee that any content on such websites is, or will remain, accurate or appropriate.

Library of Congress Cataloging-in-Publication Data

Goldsworthy, Sandra, 1961- author.
  Compact clinical guide to mechanical ventilation : foundations of practice for critical care nurses / Sandra Goldsworthy, Leslie Graham.
    p. ; cm. — (Compact clinical guide)
  Includes bibliographical references and index.
  ISBN 978-0-8261-9806-8 (alk. paper) — ISBN 0-8261-9806-6 (alk. paper) —
  ISBN 978-0-8261-9807-5 (eBook)
  I. Graham, Leslie, 1956- author. II. Title. III. Series: Compact clinical guide series.
  [DNLM: 1. Respiration, Artificial—methods. 2. Respiration, Artificial—nursing.
  3. Critical Care—methods. 4. Critical Illness—nursing. WY 163]
  RC735.I5
  615.8'362--dc23
                        2013036255

Printed in the United States of America by Gasch Printing.

This book is dedicated to all of the critical care nurses I have had the privilege to teach and mentor and to the wonderful nurses that have mentored me and provided friendship and encouragement along the way.

—Sandra

This book is dedicated to those who have taught me about mechanical ventilation educators, critical care registered nurses, and patients. I couldn't have completed this without the support of my family—thanks to each of you.

—Leslie

Contents

Foreword

As I cross the country speaking and teaching about the management of patients on ventilators, I am frequently asked, "What's out there on this topic that I can use in my practice?" What clinicians are looking for is something that may be used as a pocket reference that is concise, user friendly, and comprehensive. Although reference books do exist on the topic, few actually meet these goals, they are rarely written for nurses, and often end up on a shelf versus at the bedside.

In this book, Goldsworthy and Graham have hit the mark by providing a well-written pocket guide for critical care nurses (novice and experienced) to use as a quick reference when caring for patients requiring mechanical ventilation (MV). The content moves from oxygenation concepts and the pathophysiology of conditions that often result in the need for MV, to modes of ventilation, strategies for caring for ventilated patients, weaning (short and long term), and basic respiratory pharmacology. In keeping with the global importance of caring for our ventilated patients by applying the best available evidence, the authors also share international perspectives on the topic. Future directions for research and the development of best practices are discussed to help us consider ways to share and potentially improve clinical outcomes for our patients. Finally, each chapter provides questions and answers for the reader to test his or her understanding of the essential content.

As Goldilocks noted when she tested the bear family's three beds: "This one is too hard," "This one is too soft," but "This one is just right!" Goldsworthy and Graham have provided exactly what they intended to provide: a pocket reference that is "just right" for the bedside clinician!

Suzanne M. Burns RN, MSN, ACNP, CCRN, RRT, FAAN,
FCCM, FAANP
Professor Emeritus
School of Nursing
University of Virginia
Consultant, Critical and Progressive Care Nursing
and Clinical Nursing Research

Preface

Caring for a patient requiring mechanical ventilation in the intensive care unit can be a daunting task. Furthermore, keeping up with the latest evidence-based practice in mechanical ventilation can be a challenge, even for experienced critical care nurses.

The *Compact Clinical Guide to Mechanical Ventilation* was conceptualized as a comprehensive, practical guide for critical care nurses to use at the bedside to aid in providing high-quality patient care. This *Clinical Guide* will be useful for both the novice and experienced critical care nurse in the application of evidence-based practice at the bedside.

With many years of practice at the bedside, as clinical educators and educators in graduate critical care certificate programs, our vision is to take foundational concepts for the critical care nurse, such as mechanical ventilation, and translate them into easy-to-understand, practical information for immediate use at the bedside. Over the years of providing critical care education for registered nurses, we have both observed and been told by our students about the areas they find the most difficult to understand and apply.

Many mechanical ventilation texts are written by physicians and respiratory therapists and include explanations from their perspectives. This text is co-authored by two registered nurses who have practiced in critical care for many years as bedside practitioners and as clinical/classroom/online/simulation educators. The intent of writing this book for critical care nurses is to translate difficult concepts into understandable, manageable pieces. In this text the key components of nursing management of the patient are highlighted and described in detail. Illustrations and figures are included to help further explain mechanical ventilation. Key take-home points, case studies, and practice questions (with answers) are provided to further illustrate the main content areas. We have endeavored to include all of the tips and clinical pearls we use when teaching in our critical care practice.

This *Clinical Guide* is organized by the key concepts of critical care for the patient requiring mechanical ventilation. The first two chapters focus on oxygen therapy and a general overview of concepts, such as advanced pathophysiology, as well as indications for and complications of mechanical ventilation. In Chapter 3, the modes of ventilation and methods of providing mechanical ventilation are discussed. Chapters 4 through 7 provide the evidence-based approach to nursing management of patients requiring mechanical ventilation. Future directions are explored in Chapter 8.

We hope you will find this resource helpful at the bedside in preparing for and caring for your critically ill patients.

Sandra Goldsworthy and Leslie Graham

Acknowledgments

We want to thank Elizabeth Nieginski, Executive Editor at Springer Publishing Company, for her gracious support of this project. Through her vision, this resource for critical care nurses has become a reality. We wish to acknowledge Chris Teja, Assistant Editor, for his direction in preparing this manuscript.

1

Oxygen Delivery

In this chapter, oxygen delivery and distribution are discussed. Important aspects of respiratory physiology, neuroanatomy, and safety considerations with oxygen delivery are highlighted. In addition, common artificial airways and oxygen delivery methods are explored, focusing on the advantages, disadvantages, and nursing implications for each.

THE UPPER AND LOWER AIRWAY

Let's review! In Figure 1.1, note the components of the upper and lower airway. When a patient is mechanically ventilated and/or has an artificial airway in place, certain functions of the airway are bypassed, such as humidification and some of the airway defense mechanisms (i.e., ciliary action).

Both the upper and lower airways and alveoli have a number of defense mechanisms to guard against infection and irritation (see Table 1.1).

Patients lose their normal respiratory defense mechanisms due to the following situations:

- Disease/Illness
- Injury
- Anesthesia
- Corticosteroids
- Smoking
- Malnutrition
- Ethanol
- Uremia
- Hypoxia/Hyperoxia
- Artificial airways

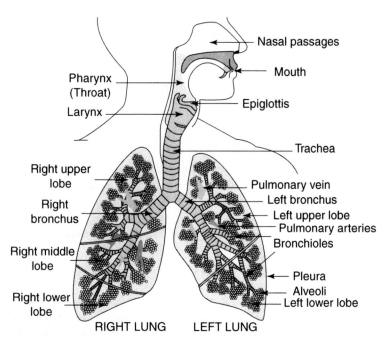

Figure 1.1 ▩ Upper and lower airways.

Table 1.1 ▩ *Pulmonary Defense Mechanisms*

Upper Airway	*Lower Airway*	*Alveoli*
• Nasal cilia	• Cough	• Immune system
• Sneeze	• Mucociliary escalator	• Lymphatics
• Cough	• Lymphatics	• Alveolar macrophages:
• Mucociliary escalator		mononuclear phago-
(mucus produced and		cytes (engulf bacteria
then propelled upward		and other foreign
by pulsatile motion and		substances)
then expectorated or		
swallowed)		
• Lymphatics		

THE PROCESS OF GAS EXCHANGE

In the pulmonary system, gas exchange occurs from the respiratory bronchioles to the alveoli. These areas receive nutrients and oxygen from the pulmonary circulation. The *acinus* refers to the terminal respiratory unit distal to the terminal bronchioles, which has an alveolar membrane for gas exchange. The respiratory bronchioles are less than 1 mm in diameter and this is where gas exchange takes place. In addition, alveolar ducts, alveolar sacs, and alveoli are lined with alveolar epithelium and this is the site where diffusion of O_2 and CO_2 between inspired air and blood occurs. Type 1 pneumocytes cover 90% of the alveolar surface and are responsible for the air–blood barrier. Type 2 pneumocytes cover 5% of the total alveolar surface and are responsible for producing and storing surfactant that lines the inner aspect of the alveolus. A deficiency of surfactant in the lungs causes alveolar collapse, loss of lung compliance, and alveolar edema. The half-life of surfactant is only 14 hours and therefore injury to the cells that produce surfactant can cause massive atelectasis (MacIntyre & Branson, 2009).

The alveolar-capillary membrane lines the respiratory bronchioles and provides a diffusion pathway where gases travel from the alveolus to the blood (O_2) or from the blood to the alveolus (CO_2). This membrane is very thin and allows for rapid gas exchange by diffusion (see Figure 1.2).

Pulmonary capillary endothelial cells have several functions:

- To produce and degrade prostaglandins
- To metabolize vasoactive amines
- To convert angiotensin I to angiotensin II
- To partly produce coagulation factor VIII

NEUROANATOMY OF THE PULMONARY SYSTEM

There are several components that are involved in the rate, rhythm, and depth of ventilation. The medulla area of the brain is responsible for controlling the central and arterial chemoreceptors. *Central chemoreceptors* are sensitive to cerebral spinal fluid pH and serve as the primary control of ventilation. Central chemoreceptors are influenced by levels of $PaCO_2$ and pH. For instance, an increase in $PaCO_2$ causes an increase in the rate and depth of ventilation, and a decrease in $PaCO_2$ causes a decrease in ventilation rate and depth.

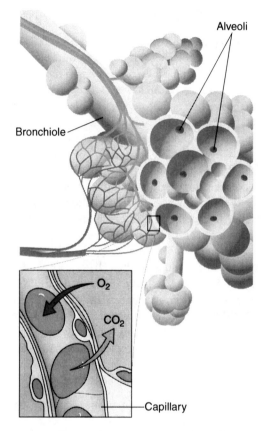

Figure 1.2 ▪ Diagram of gas exchange process and the diffusion pathway.

Arterial chemoreceptors are found within the aortic arch and carotid bodies and are sensitive to levels of pH and PaO_2. Arterial chemoreceptors provide secondary control of ventilation and respond when the PaO_2 falls below 60 mmHg.

Another area of the brain, the pons, controls the stretch receptors, proprioceptors, and baroreceptors, all of which can affect ventilation rate and rhythm. *Stretch receptors* are present in the alveoli to inhibit further inspiration and prevent overdistension. This is referred to as the "Hering–Breuer reflex." *Proprioceptors* are located in the muscles and tendons and increase ventilation in response to body movement. *Baroreceptors* are found in the aortic arch and carotid bodies and can increase blood pressure in response to cardiac output changes, which in turn can inhibit ventilation.

PHYSIOLOGY OF VENTILATION

Ventilation refers to "the movement of air between the atmosphere and the alveoli and distribution of air within the lungs to maintain appropriate levels of O_2 and CO_2 in the alveoli" (Dennison, 2013, p. 252).

The process of ventilation takes place thorough the cycle of inspiration and expiration (Table 1.2).

DEAD-SPACE VENTILATION

Alveolar ventilation refers to the volume of air per minute that is participating in gas exchange. This volume is calculated by the following equation: minute volume minus dead-space ventilation. *Dead-space ventilation* refers to the volume of air per minute that does not participate in gas exchange. There are three types of dead space: anatomic dead space, alveolar (pathologic) dead space, and physiologic dead space. *Anatomic dead space* refers to the volume of air in conducting airways that does not participate in gas exchange. Alveolar (pathologic) dead space is the volume of air in contact with nonperfused alveoli. Physiologic dead space is anatomic plus alveolar dead space (or total dead space).

Table 1.2 ▨ *Inspiration and Expiration*

Inspiration	Expiration
• Atmospheric air travels into the alveoli	• Movement of air from alveoli to atmosphere
• Message is sent from the medulla to the phrenic nerve to the diaphragm	• Relaxation of diaphragm and external intercostal muscles
• Diaphragm and intercostal muscles contract	• Recoil of lungs to resting size
• Thorax increases, lungs are stretched	• Air movement out of lungs to equalize pressure
• Air moves into lungs to equalize difference between atmospheric and alveolar pressures	

WORK OF BREATHING

The work of breathing (WOB) should be negligible; it is only responsible for 2% to 3% of the total energy expenditure of the body. If the patient is working at breathing, further assessment is required because this is not a normal finding. The WOB is related to compliance and resistance of the lungs and thorax. Compliance is a measure of expandability of the lungs and/or thorax. Factors that affect static compliance of the chest wall or lung include:

- Kyphoscoliosis
- Flail chest
- Thoracic pain with splinting
- Atelectasis
- Pneumonia
- Pulmonary edema
- Pulmonary fibrosis
- Pleural effusion
- Pneumothorax

Airway resistance can affect compliance of the lungs and can be caused by such factors as bronchospasm, mucus in airways, artificial airways, water condensation in ventilator tubing, asthma, anaphylaxis, mucosal edema, and bronchial tumor.

PERFUSION

The pulmonary system is perfused by movement of blood through the pulmonary capillaries. When a patient has decreased oxygen flow to the lungs, *hypoxic pulmonary vasoconstriction* (HPV) can occur in a localized or generalized manner. Localized pulmonary vasoconstriction is a protective mechanism in which blood flow is decreased to an area of poor ventilation so that blood can be shunted to areas of better ventilation. Localized pulmonary constriction is stimulated by alveolar O_2 levels. If all alveoli have low O_2 levels (i.e., with alveolar hypoventilation), hypoxemic pulmonary vasoconstriction may be distributed over the lungs resulting in an increased pulmonary artery pressure (PAP) and increased pulmonary vascular resistance (PVR).

VENTILATION/PERFUSION AND V/Q MISMATCH

In order for optimal gas exchange to take place from the lungs to the blood supply and onward to the tissues, a good match must be present between the perfusion (blood supply) and ventilation (gas supply). If there is a malfunction of either of these factors, then there is considered to be a "ventilation/perfusion (V/Q) mismatch" and gas exchange will not be ideal. There are three types of mismatches:

V > Q • Ventilation is acceptable but there is a problem with perfusion. • (V/Q ratio > 0.8 = high V/Q ratio)	Causes: • Pulmonary embolism • Shock • Increased tidal volume (Vt) or positive end expiratory pressure (PEEP)	**Dead-Space Unit**
Q > V • Perfusion is acceptable but there is a problem with the ventilation. • (V/Q < 0.8 = low V/Q ratio)	Causes: • Atelectasis • Acute respiratory distress syndrome (ARDS) • Pneumonia	**Shunt Unit**
No Q or V • Poor/no perfusion and ventilation	Causes: • Cardiac arrest	**Silent Unit**

Patients can also have positional V/Q mismatch because the greatest ventilation locations in the lungs are in the superior areas and the greatest perfusion areas are located in the inferior areas of the lungs. Patients can have a potential for ventilation/perfusion mismatches based on position—this is the rationale for positioning the patient with "good lung down" in unilateral lung conditions (i.e., lobectomy) to improve ventilation. This principle applies except when the patient has had a pneumonectomy.

DIFFUSION AND GAS EXCHANGE

Once ventilation and perfusion have been accounted for, the next step in gas exchange is diffusion, or movement of gases among alveoli, plasma, and the red blood cells (RBCs). General principles of diffusion include that gases move from higher to lower areas of concentration until the concentration is the same.

How Does This Happen?

During inspiration, the upper airway warms and humidifies atmospheric air as it enters the airways. As the inspired gas mixes with the gas that was not expired, the concentrations of the gases (CO_2 and O_2) change. For example, alveolar air is high in O_2 pressure and low in CO_2 pressure and the pulmonary capillary blood is high in CO_2 pressure and low in O_2 pressure. This difference in pressure causes the gases to diffuse or move across the alveolar–capillary membrane toward the lower respective pressure gradients (i.e., O_2 moves from the alveolus to the capillary and CO_2 moves from the capillary to the alveolus).

DIFFUSION DETERMINANTS

There are several factors that determine how well the diffusion of gases will occur:

- The *surface area available* for transfer (i.e., less surface area if lobectomy or pneumonectomy has occurred)
- The *thickness of the alveolar–capillary membrane* (i.e., thickened in pulmonary edema and pulmonary fibrosis making diffusion more difficult)
- The *diffusion of coefficient of gas* (i.e., CO_2 is 20 times more diffusible than O_2 so if hypoxemia is present there will be a higher likelihood of a diffusion problem than in the case of hypercapnia)
- The *driving pressure of the gas* is negatively affected by low levels of inspired oxygen (i.e., smoke inhalation or low barometric pressure as in high altitudes) and is positively affected by the addition of supplemental oxygen or higher than normal barometric pressure (i.e., hyperbaric O_2 chamber). CPAP (constant positive airway pressure) and PEEP can also increase the driving pressure of O_2.

TRANSPORT OF GASES IN THE BLOOD

Once diffusion takes place, O_2 and CO_2 move through the circulatory system. O_2 moves from the alveolus to the tissues and CO_2 moves from the tissues to the alveolus for expiration. Considerations for how well the O_2 will be transported to the cells include consideration of hemoglobin and the amount of O_2 the hemoglobin can carry (the "affinity" of hemoglobin for the O_2). The ability of the hemoglobin to transport O_2 will be negatively affected by anemia or abnormal hemoglobin (i.e., sickle cell, methoglobinemia, or carboxyhemoglobinemia). The

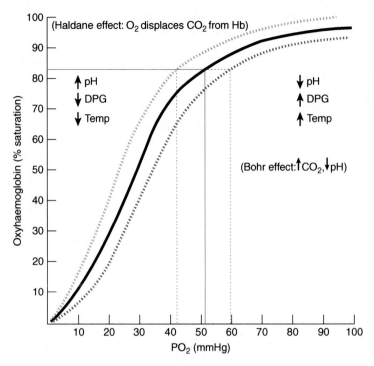

Figure 1.3 ▨ Oxyhemoglobin dissociation curve.

oxyhemoglobin dissociation curve shows the relationship between PaO$_2$ and hemoglobin saturation (Pilbeam & Cairo, 2006).

There is a substance in the erythrocyte called *2,3-DPG* that affects the affinity of hemoglobin for O$_2$. This substance is a chief end product of glucose metabolism and in the control mechanism that regulates release of O$_2$ to the tissues. When 2,3-DPG is increased, the oxyhemoglobin curve shifts to the right, decreasing affinity between hemoglobin and O$_2$. Conversely, decreased amounts of 2,3-DPG shift the curve to the left, increasing the affinity between hemoglobin and O$_2$ (see Figure 1.3 and Table 1.3).

Table 1.3 ▨ *Causes of Increased or Decreased 2,3-DPG*

Increased	Decreased
• Chronic hypoxemia	• Multiple blood transfusions
• Anemia	• Hypophosphatemia (i.e., malnutrition)
• Hyperthyroidism	• Hypothyroidism
• Pyruvate kinase deficiency	

IMPORTANT TERMS IN OXYGEN
DELIVERY AND CONSUMPTION

DO_2 (Normal = 1,000 mL/min)	The volume of O_2 *delivered* to the tissues by the left ventricle per minute
VO_2 (Normal = 250 mL/min)	The volume of O_2 *consumed* by the tissues each minute
O_2 extraction ratio	An evaluation of the amount of O_2 extracted from the arterial blood as it passes through the capillaries
Cellular respiration	The use of O_2 by the cell
SVO_2 (Normal = 60%–80%)	Provides an index of overall oxygen balance and is a reflection of the relationship between the patient's oxygen delivery (DO_2) and oxygen consumption. A change of 5% to 10% can be an early indicator of physiologic instability Factors that affect SVO_2 include: decreased O_2 delivery (i.e., decreased cardiac output, decreased hemoglobin) or increased O_2 consumption (i.e., fever, pain, seizures, numerous nursing procedures such as suctioning, chest physiotherapy)
SaO_2 (Normal = 95%–99%)	Normal levels are between 95 and 99 in a healthy individual breathing room air, levels of greater than 95 with a normal hemoglobin are acceptable range; obtained from arterial blood gas (ABG)
PaO_2 (Normal = 80–100 mmHg)	Partial pressure of arterial oxygen
SpO_2 (Normal = >95%)	Obtained from oximeter, should correlate with SaO_2
CaO_2	Oxygen content of arterial blood
PaO_2/FiO_2 ratio (Normal = 300–500)	Used to assess the severity of the gas exchange defect

There are a number of variables that affect the consumption of oxygen by the cells. The following are conditions in which there is increased oxygen consumption by the cells:

- Increased work of breathing
- Hyperthermia
- Trauma
- Sepsis

- Anxiety
- Hyperthyroidism
- Seizures/tremors

In addition there are conditions under which the cell is not able to extract, or does not require oxygen, thereby reducing oxygen consumption levels. These include:

- Hypothermia
- Sedation
- Neuromuscular blockade
- Inactivity
- Hypothyroidism
- Anesthesia

Tips for Accurate Pulse Oximetry Measurement

- Discoloration of nail bed or dark nail polish can affect transmission of light through the digit.
- Dyes used intravenously (i.e., methylene blue) can interfere with accuracy of measurement.
- Low perfusion states, such as hypotension, vasoconstriction, hypothermia, and the effects of vasoactive drips, may cause inaccurate measurement or inability to sense the SpO_2; alternate sites may have to be used (i.e., ear or forehead) rather than finger probe (Weigand-McHale, 2011).

ARTIFICIAL AIRWAYS

There are a number of circumstances in which the patient cannot protect the airway and will require the assistance of an artificial airway. In Table 1.4, a variety of common artificial airways are discussed along with potential advantages, disadvantages, and nursing implications associated with each.

Documentation: Artificial Airways

After application/insertion of an artificial airway, documentation should include the following:

- Patient and family education
- Type of airway inserted
- Size and location of airway inserted
- Respiratory assessment
- Any difficulties with insertion

- How the patient tolerated the procedure
- Vital signs and pain assessment before and after the procedure
- Verification of proper placement
- Appearance of secretions (amount, nature, color)

HYPOXEMIA AND HYPOXIA

Hypoxemia occurs when there is a decrease in arterial blood oxygen tension (i.e., a decrease in SaO_2 and PaO_2). Diagnosis of hypoxemia is made by analysis of the arterial blood gas. There are three levels of hypoxemia:

Mild hypoxemia = PaO_2 < 80 mmHg (SaO_2 < 95)
Moderate hypoxemia = PaO_2 < 60mmHg (SaO_2 < 90)
Severe hypoxemia = PaO_2 < 40mm Hg (SaO_2 < 75)

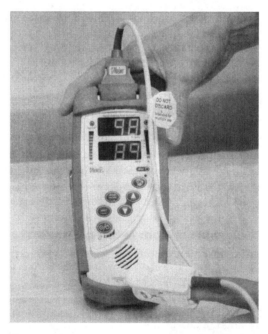

Figure 1.4 ▓ O_2 saturation (SpO_2 machine).

Table 1.4 ■ *Artificial Airways*

Artificial Airway	Advantages	Disadvantages	Nursing Care Tips and Special Notes
Oropharyngeal airway	• Quick and easy to insert • Economical • Holds tongue away from pharynx	• Easily dislodges • If incorrect size, can push tongue back and occlude airway • Not recommended in patients with head or facial trauma • Not tolerated by conscious patients, stimulates gag reflex	• Remove frequently to wash airway and provide mouth care • Use correct size (measure from edge of mouth to edge of lower lobe of ear or angle of jaw)
Nasopharyngeal ("trumpet") airway	• Quick and easy to insert • Economical • Holds tongue away from pharynx and provides air passage from the nose to pharnx • Can be used in semi-conscious or unconscious patients • Can be used when mouth cannot be opened (i.e., jaw fracture)	• Not recommended for patients on anticoagulants or at risk for nosebleeds • Can kink and clog easily • Risk of sinus infection, only use for short term	• Rotate nares to avoid nasal ulceration • Measure from tip of nose to tragas of ear

(continued)

Table 1.4 ■ *Artificial Airways* (continued)

Artificial Airway	Advantages	Disadvantages	Nursing Care Tips and Special Notes
Laryngeal Mask Airway (LMA) 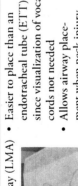	• Easier to place than an endotracheal tube (ETT) since visualization of vocal cords not needed • Allows airway placement when neck injury suspected • Permits cough and speech • Reduced risk of aspiration over mask ventilation	• Can cause laryngospasm and bronchospasm • Cannot totally prevent aspiration since GI tract and respiratory tract not separated	
Esophageal Tracheal Combitube 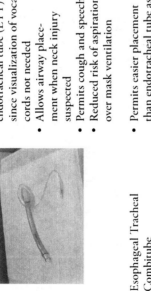 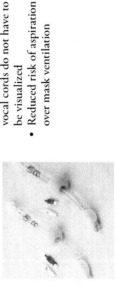 © 2013 Covidien.	• Permits easier placement than endotracheal tube as vocal cords do not have to be visualized • Reduced risk of aspiration over mask ventilation	• Cannot mechanically ventilate with combitube, long term	• Use of end tidal CO_2 recommended to confirm placement

(continued)

Table 1.4 ■ *Artificial Airways* *(continued)*

Artificial Airway	Advantages	Disadvantages	Nursing Care Tips and Special Notes
ETT (may be oral or nasal)	• Provides relatively sealed airway for mechanical ventilation • Easy to suction • Reduces risk of gastric distention • Nasal ETT more stable and patient cannot bite or chew it	• Skilled personnel required for insertion • Prevents effective cough • Loss of physiologic PEEP since epiglottis is splinted open • May have sediment build up and tube blockage (i.e., mucous plug) • Nasal ETT risk of sinus infection, cannot be used in nasal or basal skull fractures	• Rotate nares from side to side to prevent ulceration and skin breakdown • Appropriate size • Humidify and warm air • Confirm placement by x-ray, CO_2 detection device, and auscultation • Confirm cuff pressure
Tracheostomy	• Long-term airway • Minimizes vocal cord damage • Allows patient to eat and swallow • Easier suctioning • Allows effective cough • Bypasses upper airway obstruction	• Causes aphonia • May cause transcutaneous or transesophageal fistula	• Ensure correct size • Humidity needed • Keep obturator, extra tracheostomy tube and tracheal spreader at bedside

Hypoxia refers to a decrease in tissue oxygenation and is diagnosed by clinical indicators (i.e., restlessness, confusion, tachycardia, tachypnea, dyspnea, use of accessory muscles, and cyanosis). Factors that affect hypoxia include hemoglobin, SaO_2, PaO_2, cardiac output, and cellular demands (Table 1.5).

Clinical Signs of Hypoxemia/Hypoxia

Patients experiencing hypoxemia or hypoxia are often hemodynamically unstable and may have hypotension, tachycardia, arrhythmias, decreased level of consciousness, and decreased urine output. In addition, they typically have decreased PaO_2, decreased SaO_2 and decreased SVO_2 levels. Patients who are hypoxic or hypoxemic may also have increased serum lactate levels and changes in skin color and temperature.

Patients who are experiencing hypoxia or hypoxemia will typically require oxygen therapy. Indications for oxygen therapy include:

▨ Significant hypoxemia (i.e., PaO_2 < 60 mmHg)
▨ Suspected hypoxemia (pneumothorax, asthma)
▨ Increased myocardial workload (i.e., myocardial infarction)
▨ Increased oxygen demand (i.e., septic shock)
▨ Decreased oxygen's carrying capacity (i.e., anemia)
▨ Needed prior to procedures that cause hypoxia (i.e., suctioning) (Dennison, 2013, p. 295)

GENERAL PRINCIPLES OF OXYGEN THERAPY

Some general principles are important to consider when caring for a patient receiving oxygen therapy. First, to be effective an airway must be established prior to oxygen therapy. Second, oxygen is a potent drug and should only be used as needed; high concentrations of oxygen

Table 1.5 ▨ *Causes of Hypoxemia and Hypoxia*

Hypoxemia	Hypoxia
• Low inspired O_2 (high altitudes)	• Hypoxemic hypoxia (see causes under "hypoxemia")
• Hypoventilation (i.e., asthma)	
• V/Q mismatch (i.e., pulmonary embolism)	• Anemic hypoxia
• Shunt (i.e., ARDS)	• Circulatory hypoxia (i.e., shock)
• Diffusion abnormalities (i.e., pulmonary fibrosis)	• Histotoxic hypoxia (i.e., cyanide poisoning)

should be of limited duration. Third, always evaluate ABGs frequently and titrate oxygen accordingly. Remember, the objective with oxygen therapy is to improve tissue perfusion.

Clinical Pearl	**Safety Considerations: Oxygen Therapy** • No open flame or smoking near an oxygen source • Avoid petroleum-based products around O_2 • Turn off the oxygen when not in use • Secure oxygen tanks • Remove oxygen source from patient when defibrillating

HIGH-FLOW VERSUS LOW-FLOW OXYGEN DELIVERY SYSTEMS

Low-flow oxygen delivery systems (i.e., nasal cannula, simple face mask, partial rebreathing mask) are typically used when the oxygen concentration is not crucial to the patient's care. Low flow does not supply the total inspired gas; some of the patient's volume is met by breathing room air.

High-flow systems (i.e., nonrebreathing mask, Venturi mask, T-piece, tracheostomy collar, and mechanical ventilation) in contrast to low-flow systems provide a predictable fraction of inspired oxygen (FiO_2) and are more precise in the delivery of specific concentrations of oxygen.

DANGERS OF OXYGEN THERAPY

There are some hazards to be aware of in caring for patients receiving supplemental oxygen. Patients may develop oxygen-induced hypoventilation, particularly if they are chronic obstructive pulmonary disease (COPD) patients; therefore, oxygen must be carefully titrated in these patients. Patients can also develop a condition referred to as *absorptive atelectasis*. In this situation, high concentrations of O_2 wash out the nitrogen that usually holds the alveoli open at the end of expiration. It is essential to refrain from administering oxygen that is not needed in order to prevent conditions such as oxygen-induced hypoventilation and absorptive atelectasis.

Table 1.6 ■ Oxygen Delivery Methods

Oxygen Delivery Method	Advantages	Disadvantages	Nursing Implications
Nasal Cannula 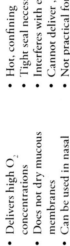 Delivers 1 to 6 L/min and 24% to 44% O_2	• Safe, simple • Good for low-flow oxygen • Economical • Allows eating, talking	• Not to be used with nasal obstruction • Drying of nasal mucosa • Skin breakdown at ears • Variable concentration of oxygen depending on tidal volume, respiratory rate, and nasal patency	• Do not exceed 6 L/min • Provide humidification if K4 L/min • Protect ears with gauze pads • Provide good oral care and moisten lips
Simple Face Mask 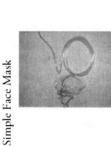 Delivers 6 to 10 L/min and 40% to 60% O_2	• Delivers high O_2 concentrations • Does not dry mucous membranes • Can be used in nasal obstruction	• Hot, confining • Tight seal necessary • Interferes with eating, talking • Cannot deliver ‹ 40% O_2 • Not practical for long term	• Pads needed to protect ears, face • Wash and dry face every 4 hours minimum • Clean mask every 8 hours and as needed • Watch for signs of O_2 toxicity

(continued)

Table 1.6 ▨ *Oxygen Delivery Methods* *(continued)*

Oxygen Delivery Method	Advantages	Disadvantages	Nursing Implications
Partial Rebreathing Mask 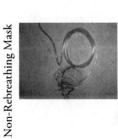 Delivers 6 to 10 L/ min. and 35% to 60% O_2	• Same as simple face mask	• Same as with other masks • May cause CO_2 retention if bag is allowed to collapse	• Ensure bag is not totally deflated • Keep mask snug • Watch for signs of O_2 toxicity
Non-Rebreathing Mask Delivers 6 to 12 L/min and 60% to 100% O_2	• One-way valve prevents rebreathing CO_2	• Same as with other masks but does not cause CO_2 retention	• Check ABGs • Watch for signs of O_2 toxicity • Ensure bag is not totally deflated

(continued)

Table 1.6 ▪ Oxygen Delivery Methods (continued)

Oxygen Delivery Method	Advantages	Disadvantages	Nursing Implications
Tracheostomy Collar 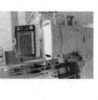 Delivers 21% to 70% O_2	• Does not pull on trach • Elastic ties allow movement of mask	• O_2 diluted by room air • Condensation can collect in tubing and drain into patient's airway	• Ensure O_2 is warmed and humidified • Empty condensation in tubing frequently
T-Piece Delivers 21% to 100% O_2	• Less moisture than trach collar • Can provide variable O_2 concentration	• May cause CO_2 retention • Can pull on tracheostomy or ETT tube	• Requires heated nebulizer • Observe for signs and symptoms of oxygen toxicity
Mechanical Ventilation 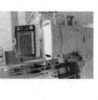 Delivers 21% to 100% O_2	• Delivers predictable, constant O_2 concentration • Can add adjuncts (i.e., PEEP) to improve ventilation	• Requires skilled personnel • Need back-up power source	• Requires heated humidifier • Need to empty condensation • Frequently assess ABGs and monitor for o2 toxicity

Adapted from Dennison (2013).

20

OXYGEN TOXICITY

When a patient receives concentrations of oxygen that are too high over too long a period of time (hours to days), oxygen toxicity can develop. Early signs and symptoms include substernal chest pain, dry cough, dyspnea, restlessness, and lethargy. Later signs of oxygen toxicity include chest x-ray changes, refractory hypoxemia, and progressive ventilator difficulty (Dennison, 2013). Oxygen toxicity may cause alveolar collapse, seizures, and retinal detachment in the eyes.

OXYGEN DELIVERY SYSTEMS

When a patient requires the administration of supplemental oxygen, a low-flow or high-flow system will be selected, in addition to a specific system for delivery and methods to evaluate the delivery's effectiveness (i.e., ABGs, continuous oximetry). Table 1.6 provides illustrations, advantages, disadvantages, and nursing implications of specific oxygen delivery methods.

Questions to Consider

The answers are found beginning on page 133.

1. Match the following with the type of V/Q mismatch: silent unit, shunt unit, dead-space unit.
   a. Pulmonary embolism
   b. Atelectasis
   c. Cardiac arrest
2. The following factors can cause decreased oxygen delivery to cells and influence SVO_2 levels. (Check all that apply.)
   _ Decreased cardiac output
   _ Fever
   _ Pain
   _ Decreased hemoglobin
   _ Anxiety
   _ Hypothermia
3. What are the early signs of oxygen toxicity?

REFERENCES

Dennison, R. (2013). *Pass CCRN!* (4th ed.). St. Louis, MO: Mosby.

MacIntyre, N., & Branson, R. (2009). *Mechanical ventilation* (2nd ed.). St. Louis, MO: Saunders.

Pilbeam, S., & Cairo, J. (2006). *Mechanical ventilation: Physiological and clinical applications*. St. Louis, MO: Mosby.

Weigand-McHale, D. (Ed.). (2011). *AACN manual for critical care*. St. Louis, MO: Elsevier.

2

Mechanical Ventilation: Overview

In this chapter an overview of mechanical ventilation is discussed. Topics include indications for mechanical ventilation, common terms, and common pathophysiology related to patients who are receiving mechanical ventilation. In addition, common equipment for mechanical ventilation is outlined (this is covered in more depth in subsequent chapters).

INDICATIONS FOR MECHANICAL VENTILATION

In order to maintain normal ventilation without supportive strategies such as mechanical ventilation, an intact rib cage and diaphragm and respiratory muscles that can contract are essential. In addition, there can be nothing interfering with intrapleural or intraalveolar pressures and the person must be able to maintain a patent airway. All of these mechanisms must be present in order to facilitate normal gas exchange.

The most common indication for mechanical ventilation is acute ventilatory failure with respiratory acidosis. Prior to ventilating a patient, underlying causes and alternative forms of maintaining ventilation must be considered because mechanical ventilation can have multiple short- and long-term complications. Other indications for mechanical ventilation are listed in Table 2.1. There are also physiologic indications that assist in the decision to mechanically ventilate the patient, including:

- Vital capacity < 10 mL/kg
- Unable to achieve maximal inspiratory force to –25 cm H_2O
- PaO_2 < 50 mmHg with an FiO_2 of >.60 (oxygenation issue)
- pH < 7.25 (ventilation issue)
- Arterial $PaCO_2$ < 30 or > 50
- Dead space/tidal volume ratio 0.6
- Respiratory rate > 35/min (Dennison, 2013)

Table 2.1 ▨ *Indications for Mechanical Ventilation*

- Acute respiratory failure
- Unable to stabilize the chest wall (i.e., trauma, flail chest, penetrating injuries)
- After major surgery to maintain oxygenation
- Cardiogenic or septic shock to decrease myocardial workload and maintain oxygenation
- Severe asthma/anaphylaxis
- Acute respiratory distress syndrome (ARDS)
- Pneumonia
- Burns and smoke inhalation
- Neuromuscular disease (i.e., Guillian-Barré, amyotrophic lateral sclerosis [ALS], myasthenia gravis)
- Overdose
- Brainstem injury
- Chronic obstructive pulmonary disease (COPD) (i.e., emphysema, cystic fibrosis)

It is essential to determine whether the underlying issue causing the respiratory failure is an oxygenation issue, a ventilation issue, or both. For a more comprehensive discussion on ventilation/perfusion mismatches, see Chapter 1. An example of a ventilation issue would include conditions that cause massive atelectasis. In this instance, the ventilation demand exceeds the ventilation supply and muscles of respiration become fatigued with increased work of breathing (WOB). This condition is also referred to as *hypercapnic failure*. In contrast, a pulmonary embolus is an example of a perfusion issue within the lungs. An oxygenation issue or *hypoxemic respiratory failure* creates a physiologic shunt in which ventilation is not interfacing with the pulmonary capillary and the patient becomes increasingly hypoxemic. In the end, if it has been determined that the patient requires mechanical ventilation, the underlying cause needs to be quickly treated and the patient's status needs to be continually reassessed to prevent complications and avoid long-term mechanical ventilation, if possible.

Prior to mechanically ventilating a patient, the patient may require intubation to protect the airway. There are a number of reasons intubation may be considered: severe acidosis or hypoxemia, severe dyspnea, respiratory arrest, cardiovascular instability, aspiration risk, copious/viscous secretions, facial trauma, and extreme obesity (Baird & Bethel, 2011). If the patient continues to deteriorate, as evidenced by the clinical presentation, arterial blood gas (ABG) trends, and other diagnostics such as chest x-ray, in addition to being unable to quickly treat the underlying cause, mechanical ventilation may be required.

COMMON TERMS

There are a number of common terms with which the nurse needs to be familiar in order to care for a patient who is receiving mechanical ventilation. Knowledge of these terms will aid the registered nurse in accurately documenting changes in the patient's progress and will also provide a common language when discussing mechanical ventilation with other health care team members.

Respiratory Rate (RR): This refers to the number of breaths per minute taken by the patient or delivered by the ventilator. It is important to distinguish the number of spontaneous breaths from the number of machine-delivered breaths to determine the patient's underlying respiratory effort. Normal spontaneous respiratory rate is 12 to 20 breaths per minute. Ventilator-delivered respiratory rate can vary from 10 to 50 breaths per minute (except during weaning when the rate may be less than 10) depending on the goal and strategies of the treatment and the patient's spontaneous effort.

Tidal Volume (V_T): This is the amount of gas delivered with each preset breath by the ventilator or volume of breath spontaneously taken by the patient. Mechanical ventilator-set tidal volume is usually no greater than 8 to 10 mL/kg to avoid barotrauma and long-term complications. The set tidal volume may be lower (i.e., 6–8 mL/kg) in patients with noncompliant lungs (Baird & Bethel, 2011).

Minute Volume (V_E): The minute volume refers to the amount of lung volume exhaled in 1 minute. Normal lung volume is 8 to 10 L/min.

Fraction of Inspired Oxygen (FiO_2): This refers to the percentage of atmospheric pressure that is oxygen (see Chapter 1 for an in-depth description of oxygenation).

Peak Inspiratory Pressure (PIP): This is the peak pressure measured as each ventilator breath is given. To guard against barotrauma, high and low-pressure alarms are set in relation to the PIP. Normal PIP is less than 35 cm H_2O. If resistance increases in the lungs or lung compliance decreases as a result of a pathologic condition (i.e., ARDS), the PIP will increase. If there is a disconnection or leak in the ventilator circuit, the PIP will sound an alarm indicating a low value.

Mean Airway Pressure (MAP): The MAP refers to the average pressure in the airway over the entire respiratory cycle. If the pressures remain too high, alternative ventilation strategies may need to be explored.

Flow Rate (V): The flow rate is the method and rate for the tidal volume to be delivered by the mechanical ventilator with each breath. Normal is 40 to 100 L/min. The flow rate may be manipulated to change time spent in inspiration or expiration.

Trigger: The trigger function is set to to cause the desired inspiratory flow from the ventilator. For instance, the breath can be "triggered" by either elapsed time (i.e., to a set number of breaths in a minute) or to the patient's negative inspiratory force (respiratory effort). In this mode, the patient's breath can be sensed as a change of flow in the circuit and it can allow the spontaneous breath to occur.

Sensitivity: This setting adjusts how much effort the patient must generate (negative inspiratory force) before the ventilator delivers a breath. This setting is only activated in the assist/control or SIMV (synchronized intermittent mandatory ventilation) modes (see Chapter 3 for a detailed discussion of ventilator modes.

Cycle: The "cycle" is the opposite of a trigger. *Cycle* refers to what stops the inspiratory flow or stops the breath delivery by the ventilator.

1. **Pressure Cycle**
   In a pressure cycle breath, a predetermined and preset pressure terminates inspiration. In this mode, pressure is constant and volume is variable depending on the compliance of the lungs.

2. **Volume Cycle**
   In a volume-cycle breath, a predetermined volume will terminate the respiration once delivered.

3. **Time Cycle**
   Time cycle refers to air/gas being delivered over a preset time frame. This mode effects the inspiration to expiration (I:E) ratio. A time-cycle breath is directly related to how quickly or slowly the tidal volume occurs.

PATHOPHYSIOLOGY

The following are highlights of the key conditions that may require the patient to be mechanically ventilated.

Acute Respiratory Failure

Pathophysiology

In acute respiratory failure, the patient is unable to maintain the acid–base balance and the normal exchange of carbon dioxide and oxygen. Typically, the patient's deterioration is reflected in the blood gas results, which demonstrate a PaO_2 of less than 60, an FiO_2 of greater than 0.50, and a pH of less than 7.25. If the underlying cause is not reversed, the patient eventually tires and cannot maintain respiratory effort.

There are four main pathophysiologic causes of acute respiratory failure: hypoventilation, ventilation/perfusion (V/Q) mismatching, shunting, and diffusion effects. In the case of hypoventilation, the patient retains carbon dioxide and becomes hypoxemic. Causes of hypoventilation are damage to or depression of the neurologic system (e.g., head injury, cerebral thrombosis, or hemorrhage), neuromuscular defects causing hypoventilation (e.g., myasthenia gravis, multiple sclerosis, Guillian–Barré syndrome), obstructive lung conditions (e.g., asthma, emphysema, and cystic fibrosis), and restrictive lung conditions (e.g., obesity, flail chest, lung cancer, and pneumothorax).

V/Q mismatching is another potential cause of acute respiratory failure. Ventilation abnormalities can occur in asthma, pneumonia, and when tumors are present, whereas perfusion abnormalities can occur with pulmonary embolism, excessive positive end expiratory pressure (PEEP), and decreased cardiac output. When there are V/Q mismatches present, such as when perfusion is greater than ventilation or vice versa, hypoxemia results.

The third category of acute respiratory failure is the development of a shunt. When blood bypasses the alveolar–capillary unit (anatomic shunt) or blood goes through the alveolar–capillary unit but it is nonfunctional (physiologic shunt), oxygenation does not take place. Examples of anatomic shunts include arteriovenous (AV) shunts and shunts associated with neoplasms. Physiologic shunt examples include atelectasis, pneumothorax, pneumonias, cardiac pulmonary edema, and near drowning.

Lastly, diffusion abnormalities can cause acute respiratory failure. Increased diffusion pathways can occur with accumulation of fluid, such as with pulmonary edema and pulmonary fibrosis. Decreased diffusion areas can occur with surgical procedures such as a lobectomy as well as with destructive lung diseases such as emphysema and tumors. All of these mechanisms will precipitate acute respiratory failure and hypoxemia and must be treated.

Clinical Manifestations

Key signs and symptoms of acute respiratory failure include increased respiratory rate with decreased tidal volume (i.e., rapid, shallow breaths), increase in WOB with accessory muscle use, complaints of dyspnea, hypoxemia (decreased SpO_2 and PaO_2), hypercapnia, anxiety, and restlessness.

Management

Treatment of acute respiratory failure is aimed at improving oxygenation through measures such as treating the cause, oxygen delivery, positioning, bronchial hygiene, pharmacological therapy, and, potentially, mechanical ventilation if the patient's condition deteriorates. It is essential that the nurse and health care team closely monitor the patient's changing status, watching for clinical signs of deterioration and downward trends in arterial blood gas and chest x-ray results. In addition, adequate hydration is required and a quiet, restful environment without overstimulation is essential.

Complications

The nurse should monitor for complications of acute respiratory failure, which could include:

- Arrhythmias
- Pneumonia
- Pulmonary edema
- Pulmonary embolism
- Pulmonary fibrosis
- Oxygen toxicity
- Renal failure
- Acid–base imbalance
- Electrolyte imbalance
- Gastrointestinal complications (e.g., ulceration, hemorrhage)
- Disseminated intravascular coagulation (DIC)
- Septic shock
- Delirium

ARDS

Pathophysiology

ARDS has an acute onset and demonstrates bilateral lung opacities with pulmonary edema on the chest x-ray. There are three categories of ARDS: mild, moderate, and severe (Table 2.2). ARDS results from

Table 2.2 ▦ *ARDS Severity*

	PaO$_2$/FiO$_2$ Ratio	*Mortality Rates*
Mild (previously called acute lung injury [ALI])	200–300	27%
Moderate	100–200	32%
Severe	< 100	45%

From ARDS Definition Task Force (2012).

direct (i.e. pneumonia, aspiration, lung contusions, inhalation/burn injury, severe acute respiratory syndrome [SARS]) or indirect lung injury (i.e., severe sepsis, trauma, pancreatitis, transfusion-related lung injury [TRALI] or ventilator-associated lung injury [VALI]) and can have a mortality rate of more than 60%.

Once the lungs have sustained an indirect or direct injury, mediators are released that cause increasing vascular and capillary permeability (leaking). This leads to alveolar collapse and accumulation of fluids in the pulmonary interstitium. As the condition worsens, surfactant production is decreased, protein production increases, and gas exchange decreases. Initially, hypoxemia develops and then worsens, leading to eventual hypercapnic respiratory failure. Shunt and dead space increase and lead to noncompliant, stiff lungs with derecruited alveoli. Diffuse pulmonary infiltrates and refractory hypoxemic respiratory failure define the exacerbated process of ARDS, which still, despite aggressive treatment and advances in this area, leads to high mortality rates.

Clinical Manifestations
The clinical presentation of ARDS is given in Table 2.3.

Table 2.3 ▦ *ARDS*

Initially	*Ventilator Pressures*
• Cyanosis	• Increasing peak and plateau pressures
• Pallor	• PaO$_2$/FIO$_2$ ratio declines further
• Accessory muscle use	
• Tachypnea	
• Tachycardia	
• Diaphoresis	
• Decreased level of consciousness	
• Decreased bronchial breath sounds	

Management

Diagnostic tests used in ARDS include pulmonary function studies, arterial blood gas analysis, complete blood count (CBC), coagulation profiles, tracheal–protein/plasma–protein ratio, and chest x-ray. Management of ARDS is aimed at determining and treating the underlying cause. Supportive measures include oxygen therapy, mechanical ventilation with moderate to high levels of PEEP, low tidal volumes, and patient positioning. Repositioning the patient at least every 2 hours (more often if possible) is best. The use of continuous lateral motion therapy beds or prone positioning can be very beneficial to the patient with ARDS. Repositioning techniques assist by redistributing the interstitial edema with the goal of improving oxygenation. Other treatment management includes maintaining adequate hydration, appropriate sedation (see Chapter 7), and nutritional support to maintain energy needed for healing. Continuous monitoring and reassessment of the patient are required since the patient's condition can change and worsen very rapidly. Mechanical ventilation strategies may vary in ARDS depending on the stage of the disease and the patient response. Permissive hypercapnia, inverse ratio ventilation, high-frequency oscillation, and inhaled nitric oxide and recruitment maneuvers such as high levels of PEEP may be used in an attempt to improve patient outcomes. There are three stages to the progression and potential resolution of ARDS. The first phase lasts approximately 1 week, followed by the proliferative phase, which lasts 7 to 14 days. The last stage is the fibrotic stage, which resolves very slowly (Carlson, 2009). In summary, key management of ARDS includes lower tidal volumes, PEEP, conservative fluid therapy, and refraining from using pulmonary artery catheters for routine management (Saguil & Fargo, 2012).

Complications

If there is resolution of ARDS, long-term complications can include persistent restrictive and obstructive pulmonary deficits, bronchial hyperactivity, and posttraumatic stress disorder (common in survivors). ARDS survivors can also experience long-term significant weakness from neuropathy and myopathy (Griffiths & Hall, 2010) in addition to persistent cognitive impairment (Herridge, Tansey, & Matte, 2011; Iwashyna, Ely, Smith, & Langa, 2010).

Pneumonia

Pathophysiology

Pneumonia is an acute infection that causes inflammation of the alveolar spaces and lung tissue. It is one of the leading causes of death in North America (Bethel & Baird, 2011). There are several classifications of pneumonia: community acquired, hospital acquired or nosocomial, aspiration pneumonia, and ventilator-associated pneumonia (VAP). Community-acquired pneumonia refers to a pneumonia that has been acquired outside of the hospital, whereas nosocomial pneumonia occurs while in hospital and is the most likely to be lethal to patients. Aspiration pneumonia results from aspiration of the oropharyngeal or gastric contents and can result in ARDS. VAP refers to a patient who has acquired pneumonia more than 48 hours after endotracheal intubation and mechanical ventilation. See Chapter 4 for a more complete discussion of the prevention of VAP.

Clinical Manifestations

Clinical presentation of pneumonia includes the following:

- A persistent cough that may or may not be productive
- Sputum presence depending on the pathogen
- Pleuritic chest pain
- Chest x-ray showing infiltrates
- Fever
- Decreased SpO_2
- Tachycardia and tachypnea
- May be hypotensive if septic
- Respiratory distress with use of accessory muscles
- Cyanosis
- Ashen or pale appearance
- Anxiety, agitation
- Decreased breath sounds
- Crackles on inspiration

Management

Close assessment of changing respiratory status is required by the nurse. In addition, monitoring of a number of diagnostic tests may assist in determining the underlying cause and patient status. Diagnostic tests include ABGs, CBC, sputum cultures, blood cultures, chest x-rays, and potential bronchoscopy or thoracentesis.

Priorities in patient management of pneumonia include treating hypoxemia, controlling the infection with antibiotics, anti-infectives, cough control, adequate hydration, pain assessment and treatment, nutrition, and bronchial hygiene to relieve congestion. In addition, elevating the head of the bed prevents VAP and promotes ventilation, peptic ulcer prevention, and mobility and range-of-motion exercises.

Complications

Complications of pneumonia include sepsis, septic shock, and respiratory failure, which can involve high rates of mortality.

Asthma

Pathophysiology

In asthma, airway narrowing occurs as a result of an extrinsic trigger causing immunoglobulin E (IgE) to be released. Common triggers of asthma are respiratory infections, allergens, smoke, exercise, and extreme anxiety. Inflammation and bronchoconstriction occur as a result, with trapped air causing hyperinflation of the alveoli. In addition, an increased amount of thick mucus is secreted as a result of histamine release. This inflammation, narrowed airway, and mucus production causes V/Q mismatch and hypoxemia, which will result in acute respiratory failure if not treated quickly.

Clinical Manifestations

The patient experiencing asthma typically presents with the following symptoms: anxiety, dyspnea, chest tightness, fatigue, diaphoresis, dehydration (especially mucous membranes), anorexia, tachycardia, tachypnea, and productive cough. In addition, the patient exhibits signs and symptoms of respiratory distress, such as the use of accessory muscles, nasal flaring, increased WOB, and wheezing heard bilaterally.

Management

Priorities in caring for the patient experiencing severe asthma include determining the severity of asthma, oxygen therapy, and pharmacological treatment. The main objective is to treat the bronchospasm and prevent further hypoxemia. Aggressive therapy is required to reduce severe asthma and requires bronchodilators, corticosteroids, and anticholinergics (to reduce vagal tone of the airway). In addition, antibiotics may be required to treat any underlying respiratory infection. Fluid replacement will be needed to treat dehydration. Other supportive care includes vigorous chest physiotherapy and bronchial hygiene to promote release of secretions. The nurse will need to closely monitor the patient's changing respiratory status and vital signs, as well as assess the results of ABGs, CBC, and electrolyte blood work. The patient experiencing severe asthma will be very anxious and it is important to explain procedures; provide reassurance; enable family members to stay with the patient; and maintain a restful, quiet environment.

Complications
As asthma worsens, the patient can become exhausted, resulting in an increasingly weak respiratory effort leading to further decreased breath sounds, bradycardia, cyanosis, hypotension, arrhythmias, coma, and respiratory arrest. If the patient develops life-threatening complications, mechanical ventilation may be required.

EQUIPMENT

The equipment required to mechanically ventilate (see Figure 2.1) a patient involves three overall functions that include power input, a control scheme, and an output mechanism (MacIntyre & Branson, 2009).

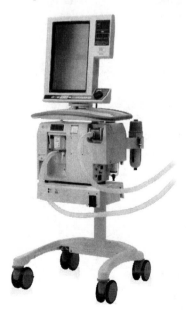

Figure 2.1 ■ Ventilator.
Source: Trademark of Covidien AG or its affiliates. © 2013 Covidien.

First, the source of power is needed, with the most commonly used types being electric (to operate the control circuit) and pneumatic/compressed gas to provide the energy to ventilate the lungs. The second function required of the ventilator is the control scheme. The control scheme manages the pressure, volume, flow, and time of the mechanically ventilated breaths. Finally, the output function of the ventilator provides waveforms (i.e., for pressure, volume, and flow), as well as a display that allows the nurse to monitor and document settings and patient response to ventilation. In addition to the mechanical ventilator machine, associated ventilator tubing and humidifiers are required to complete the circuit and provide ventilation through the endotracheal tube (ETT) or alternate airway (see Chapter 1 for a further description of airways).

SUMMARY

In this chapter, common terms used in ventilation were discussed in addition to common types of pathophysiology and indications for mechanical ventilation. The clinical presentation and key management features of acute respiratory failure, ARDS, pneumonia, and asthma were presented.

Questions to Consider

The answers are found beginning on page 133.

1. List five potential indications for mechanical ventilation.
2. What are the physiologic indications for mechanical ventilation?
3. What are the classifications of ARDS and associated PaO_2/FiO_2 ratios?
4. Long-term complications of ARDS can include persistent muscle weakness, posttraumatic stress disorder, and cognitive impairment.
   a. True
   b. False
5. Normal PIPs are:
   a. < 50 cm H_2O
   b. < 35 cm H_2O
   c. < 15 cm H_2O

Case Study

Ms. Woodgate, 22 years old, is admitted to the emergency department with acute exacerbation of asthma. Her vital signs are:

Heart rate (HR) 118, sinus tachycardia
RR 30/min
SpO_2 91%
Blood pressure (B/P) 102/66

She has wheezing bilaterally, with decreased breath sounds to both lung bases. Ms. Woodgate is very anxious and diaphoretic; her oral mucous membranes are dry and she says it is very difficult to breathe. Despite treatment with oxygen, bronchodilators, and steroids, her condition continues to worsen.

1. What are common triggers for asthma exacerbations?
2. The goal of treatment with Ms. Woodgate is to treat _____ and prevent _____.
3. Provide examples of supportive treatment required in the treatment of Ms. Woodgate's acute exacerbation of asthma.

REFERENCES

ARDS Definition Task Force. (2012). Acute respiratory distress syndrome: The Berlin definition. *Journal of the American Medical Association, 307*(23), 2526–2533.

Baird, M., & Bethel, S. (2011). *Manual of critical care nursing: Nursing interventions and collaborative management* (6th ed.). St. Louis, MO: Elsevier.

Carlson, K. (Ed.). (2009). *Advanced critical care nursing.* St. Louis, MO: Saunders.

Dennison, R. (2013). *Pass CCRN!* (4th ed). St. Louis, MO: Mosby.

Griffiths, R., & Hall, J. (2010). Intensive care acquired weakness. *Critical Care Medicine, 38*(3), 779–787.

Herridge, M., Tansey, C., & Matté, A. (2011). Canadian Critical Care Trials Group. Functional disability 5 years after acute respiratory distress syndrome. *New England Journal of Medicine, 364*(14), 1293–1304.

Iwashyna, T., Ely, E., Smith, D., & Langa, K. (2010). Long-term cognitive impairment and functional disability among survivors of severe sepsis. *Journal of the American Medical Association, 304*(16), 1787–1794.

MacIntyre, N., & Branson, R. (2009). *Mechanical ventilation* (2nd ed.). St. Louis, MO: Saunders.

Morton, P., & Fontaine, D. (2009). *Critical care cursing: A holistic approach* (9th ed.). Philadelphia, PA: Lippincott Williams and Wilkins.

Pierce, L. (2007). *Management of the mechanically ventilated patie*nt (2nd ed.). St. Louis, MO: Saunders.

Pilbeam, S., & Cairo, J. (2006*). Mechanical ventilation: Physiological and clinical applications* (4th ed.). St. Louis, MO: Mosby.

Saguil, A., & Fargo, M. (2012). ARDS treatment and management. *American Family Physician, 85*(4), 352–359.

3

Modes of Mechanical Ventilation

Mechanical ventilators have evolved significantly over the past 50 years. Early ventilators, such as the iron lung, had very simplistic modes to support the patient with respiratory failure. Ventilators and ventilation modes have continued to advance based on available research and the rapid expansion in technology (Kacmarek, 2011). This chapter explores common modes of ventilation, from basic to advanced. In addition, trouble-shooting tips are discussed.

COMMON MODES OF VENTILATION

The most common reason for initiating mechanical ventilation is respiratory failure. Respiratory failure is defined as pH less than 7.25, PaO_2 less than 60 mmHg with supplemental oxygen at greater than 50%, and $PaCO_2$ greater than 50 mmHg (Burns, 2009; Morton & Fontaine, 2013; Sole, Klein, & Moseley, 2013). In addition to worsening arterial blood gases (ABGs), the patient may also demonstrate clinical signs of deterioration. These signs include rapid shallow breathing, increased work of breathing (WOB), use of accessory muscles, and hemodynamic instability (see Chapters 2 and 4). The patient is then supported on mechanical ventilation while the underlying cause of the respiratory failure is corrected.

Modern ventilators offer a variety of modes to select from. When determining the most effective ventilation mode, the emphasis is on patient comfort and safety. In promoting lung-protective strategies, choosing the most appropriate mode will aid in prevention of *volutrauma* and *barotrauma*. The five basic modes (MacIntyre, 2011) include:

- Volume control
- Volume assist
- Pressure control
- Pressure assist
- Pressure support

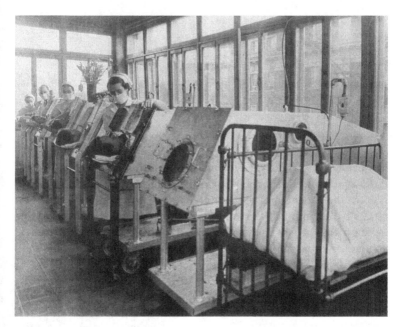

Figure 3.1 ▪ ICU with patients receiving mechanical ventilation via an iron lung. *Source:* Reprinted by permission from the hospital archives, the Hospital for Sick Children, Toronto.

The advantages and disadvantages of each of the modes are discussed in detail.

Pressure-Control Mode

Pressure-targeted ventilation is a mode in which the volume of gas is delivered until the preset pressure has been reached. In this mode, the breaths are triggered by the patient and this mode may be used independently or in conjunction with other modes. The patient may receive a variable tidal volume (V_T), depending on lung compliance, as well as airway and circuit compliance. Two of the most common pressure-targeted modes are pressure-support (PS) and pressure-control (PC) ventilation.

With PS ventilation, the patient's spontaneous breaths are augmented with a preset amount of inspiratory pressure. To use this mode, the patient's respiratory drive must be intact in order for the patient to initiate spontaneous breaths. Through the use of PS, resistance of the artificial airway and ventilator circuit is negated, resulting in decreased work of breathing. The main parameters for the clinician to set are the pressure-support level, sensitivity, FiO_2, and positive end expiratory pressure (PEEP). When high levels of PS are required, this is considered to be full ventilator support. This mode is also used in conjunction with other modes to supplement spontaneous breaths, as with synchronized intermittent mandatory ventilation (SIMV). The main advantage of this mode is the control the patient has over the ventilatory process.

Pressure-control ventilation is the mode in which a respiratory rate is set and every breath is augmented by a preset amount of inspiratory pressure. Once triggered, the gas is delivered until the preset pressure is reached. If the patient takes spontaneous breaths, those breaths are also augmented by the preset inspiratory pressure. The clinician must set the inspiratory-pressure limit, respiratory rate, inspiratory time, sensitivity, FiO_2, and PEEP. This mode is useful as a lung-protective strategy for the patient with low lung compliance, such as acute respiratory distress syndrome (ARDS) (Grossbach, Chlan, & Tracy, 2011; Kane & York, 2012). This mode is useful in controlling high-plateau pressures, which prevents the patient from developing barotrauma.

Another pressure-controlled mode is inverse-ratio ventilation. This mode is useful when the patient has poor oxygenation despite high FiO_2, PEEP, and positioning. The clinician sets the rate, sensitivity, FiO_2, and PEEP. The inspiratory time is set to provide a longer period of time in order to improve oxygenation. As this is uncomfortable for the patient, sedation and possibly paralytics are required to prevent patient-ventilator dyssynchrony and desaturation.

Airway pressure-release ventilation is often used as a lung recruitment strategy for patients who do not respond to other modes of ventilation. In this mode, there are two levels of constant positive-airway pressure (CPAP), one during inspiration and one during expiration. The patient is permitted to breath spontaneously. To initiate this mode, the clinician must set one level of relatively high CPAP, which releases after a short period of time, for a second level of CPAP during the expiratory phase. This mode is useful in decreasing airway pressure in patients with chronic obstructive pulmonary disease (COPD), trauma, and ARDS. This mode is tolerated well by patients and has the added benefit of decreasing the need for deep sedation or paralytics.

Volume-Control Mode

In volume-targeted ventilation, the V_T remains constant for each breath delivered by the ventilator. The V_T is preset and is delivered by the ventilator until the preset volume is reached. In this mode the ventilator performs all of the WOB, without the patient initiating any effort. The minute volume is entirely delivered by the ventilator. This mode is useful when the patient is experiencing apnea, for example, if the patient is suffering from a neurological condition or a drug overdose. Another reason to initiate volume-targeted ventilation is to fully rest the patient's diaphragm and respiratory muscles to allow healing of the underlying respiratory condition. To promote patient comfort, the sensitivity dial is set at −1 to −2 cm to permit the patient to trigger a ventilator breath with little effort. Conversely, this mode can also increase the WOB, create anxiety, and shortness of breath if the patient is attempting to initiate a breath and the flow rate does not match inspiratory efforts. This requires immediate alteration of the flow-rate setting (Grossbach, Chlan, & Tracy, 2011).

An example of this volume-targeted mode is assist/control ventilation (A/C). To ventilate the patient requiring A/C ventilation, the respiratory rate, V_T, sensitivity, FiO_2, and PEEP need to be set by the clinician. The patient may initiate a breath, which will be delivered at the preset V_T. Another volume-targeted mode of ventilation is SIMV. Similar to the A/C mode, in SIMV the patient will receive a preset V_T at a preset rate. The patient may initiate spontaneous breaths above the preset rate, at the patient's own spontaneous V_T. For this mode the clinician needs to set the rate, V_T, sensitivity, FiO_2, and PEEP. This mode is helpful for the patient with an intact respiratory drive but with weakened respiratory muscles. SIMV is often related to PS. PS will provide extra assistance with spontaneous breaths. In the past this mode was used as a method of weaning, gradually turning down the V_T rate of preset breaths, to allow the patient to take over the WOB. Research has shown that this method of weaning takes a long time to liberate the patient from the ventilator, which contributes to lower success rates (Pierce, 2007).

HIGH-FREQUENCY OSCILLATORY VENTILATION

High-frequency oscillatatory ventilation (HFOV) is a type of ventilation known as a rescue mode for a patient experiencing refractory hypoxemia. This mode of ventilation delivers small V_T at a rapid rate of

Table 3.1 ▦ *Advantages and Disadvantages of Ventilator Modes*

Mode	Description	Advantages	Disadvantages	Nursing Implications
Assist/Control	Used as an initial mode of ventilation or when the patient is apneic from a neurological injury	• The same V_T is delivered without reliance on lung compliance or resistance	• The patient may require sedation and paralytics to maintain this mode • May promote respiratory muscle weakness • Monitor for respiratory alkalosis due to hyperventilation	• Work of breathing may be increased if sensitivity is set inappropriately • Monitor the respiratory rate to assess patient-initiated breaths • Monitor peak inspiratory pressure to determine alterations in compliance and resistance • Assess patient comfort with setting and ABGs
SIMV	The ventilator delivers preset V_T at a preset rate, allowing the patient to initiate a spontaneous breath between mandatory breaths	• Prevents respiratory muscle weakness • Decreases risk of hyperventilation • Guarantees volume with each breath	• May develop patient–ventilator dyssynchrony due to stacking of the breaths, as a mandatory breath is delivered on top of the patient's spontaneous breath, which may lead to barotrauma	• Monitor patient's respiratory rate and spontaneous V_T • Assess for fatigue and increased work of breathing • Observe for patient–ventilator dyssynchrony; provide sedation that will not affect respiratory drive

(continued)

41

Table 3.1 ▨ *Advantages and Disadvantages of Ventilator Modes* (*continued*)

Mode	Description	Advantages	Disadvantages	Nursing Implications
Pressure support	The patient's spontaneous breaths are augmented by a preset inspiratory pressure	• Decreased O_2 consumption as a result of decreased work of breathing Improves patient comfort and patient-ventilator synchrony	• Contraindicated in patients with acute bronchospasm/copious secretions or with alteration in level of consciousness and decreased respiratory drive	• Monitor exhaled V_T and increase PS if inadequate • Monitor respiratory rate • Assess for signs of fatigue
Pressure control	A breath can be initiated by the patient or the ventilator and the gas flow is delivered at a preset pressure	• Reduces the risk of barotraumas while maintaining oxygenation and ventilation	• Patient–ventilator dyssynchrony requiring sedation/paralytics	• Monitor exhaled V_T and minute volume for any cause of increased airway resistance • Be familiar with ventilator settings, such as inspiratory pressure level • Monitor for increased respiratory rate and sedate patient as necessary or consider switching to another mode that permits spontaneous breathing • Monitor hemodynamic status as increased airway pressure may compromise venous return

(*continued*)

Table 3.1 ▓ *Advantages and Disadvantages of Ventilator Modes* *(continued)*

Mode	Description	Advantages	Disadvantages	Nursing Implications
Pressure-controlled inverse-ratio ventilation	The patient is maintained on pressure-controlled ventilation with a longer inspiratory time	This mode promotes recruitment of alveoli and improves oxygenation	Is uncomfortable for the patient and requires sedation and paralytics	• The patient must be sedated to prevent interruption of the cycle, causing loss of PEEP and alveolar collapse
Airway-pressure-release ventilation	This mode promotes lower airway pressures with improved ventilation-perfusion	This mode improves oxygenation and minimizes atelectrauma	Potential for de-recruitment of the lung if the release time is not adjusted when the lung mechanics change Difficult to auscultate breath sounds due to the short release interval	• Monitor minute ventilation, spontaneous V_T and release volumes • Respiratory rate should be counted for a full minute
PEEP or CPAP	Addition of positive pressure into the airways at the end of expiration prevents collapse of alveoli PEEP = intubated and ventilated patients CPAP = patients who breath spontaneously	This mode improves oxygenation and promotes alveolar recruitment Promotes reduction in FiO_2 to prevent oxygen toxicity	May cause an increase in intrathoracic pressure, which causes a decrease in cardiac output, volutrauma, or barotrauma	• Monitor for adequate intravascular volume and administer volume as needed or inotropes as required

Sources: Grossbach (2008); Haas and Bauser (2012); Kane and York (2012); Morron and Fontaine (2013); Pierce (2007, 2013); Sole, Klein, and Moseley (2013).

43

300 to 400 breaths per minute. The ventilator delivers this high rate with a high-frequency oscillation known as a hertz. This creates a wave or an oscillation that promotes the elimination of carbon dioxide and improves oxygenation by preventing alveolar collapse (Bortolotto & Makic, 2012; Haas & Bauser, 2012). This mode diminishes the phenomenon known as "stacking of breaths" during exhalation. When the breath is not fully exhaled, air is trapped in the noncompliant lung, which is known as auto PEEP. Auto PEEP can cause increased intrathoracic pressures, leading to a decrease in cardiac output, or barotrauma. This mode of ventilation requires a special ventilator that uses a piston to drive the gas flow in and out of the lung. The clinician needs to set mean airway pressure, frequency, inspiratory time, oscillatory pressure, and FiO_2. Complications associated with this mode of ventilation are:

- Hypotension resulting from high mean airway pressures
- Pneumothorax, which is observed when there is loss of chest wiggle on the affected side
- Endotracheal tube obstruction, with a sudden rise in carbon dioxide levels, as noted in the ABG result
- Mechanical oscillator failure (when the circuit is malfunctioning); the patient will require manual ventilation with a resuscitative bag equipped with a PEEP valve (Pierce, 2007)

NONINVASIVE VENTILATION

Noninvasive ventilation is a form of ventilation that does not use an artificial airway. This is accomplished through a tight-fitting mask that covers the mouth and nose, or with nasal prongs. This mode of ventilation—noninvasive bilateral positive pressure (BiPAP) ventilation—is especially useful for patients with pulmonary edema, early respiratory failure, and/or obstructive sleep apnea (Morton & Fontaine, 2013). Contraindications to this mode are claustrophobia, thick or copious secretions, or recent facial or gastroesophageal surgery. The clinician sets the following settings when initiating this mode of ventilation: inspiratory pressure support level, expiratory pressure, and rate of flow. Nursing management for this mode of ventilation includes:

- Correct mask size
- Assess skin under mask, straps, and across the bridge of the nose for signs of breakdown; the patient may require special wound-care products to protect the skin

- Use of nasal mask or chin strap if the patient is a mouth breather
- Access for irritated eyes caused by gases escaping around the mask; may require lubricating eye drops
- Access for dry oral mucosa; may necessitate the use of external humidification and diligent oral care
- Because the patient can eat with this mode, exercise caution to prevent aspiration

Ventilator Settings

The ventilator should be checked according to agency policy, as well as whenever changes are noted to the patient's condition. This is performed as often as every 1 to 4 hours. Depending on the jurisdiction, this duty may be shared between the registered nurse and the registered respiratory therapist. The nurse responsible for the patient needs to be aware of the alarm-level settings.

The settings the nurse needs to be familiar with:

- V_T is the volume of gas delivered with each breath. Usually this is set at 6 to 8 mL/kg ideal body weight (Sole, Klein, & Moseley, 2013). When monitoring V_T it is important to monitor the peak inspiratory pressure and reduce the V_T if the pressures are nearing 40 cm.
- **FiO$_2$** is set from 0.21 to 1.0 to maintain the patient's PaO$_2$ greater than 60 mmHg and a SaO$_2$ of at least 90%, according to the ABG values.
- **Respiratory rate** is the frequency of breath delivered by the ventilator. This may be changed frequently, depending on the patient's WOB, comfort level, pH, and PaCO$_2$.
- **PEEP** is set between 5 and 20 cm H$_2$O to prevent alveolar collapse. Monitor the patient's hemodynamic status when increasing the level of PEEP, as this may decrease venous return.
- **Sensitivity** is set to make the ventilator sensitive to the patient's inspiratory effort. If set too high, patient–ventilator dyssynchrony may occur. If set too low, this will increase the work of breathing when the patient attempts to initiate a breath.
- **Inspiratory-to-expiratory ratio** or I:E ratio needs to be set to mimic the respiratory cycle at 1:2. This can be altered to prolong the expiratory phase for patients with COPD (Grossbach, 2008).

Data that the nurse is required to assess:

- Minute volume, which is the volume of gas exhaled in 1 minute
- Exhaled V_T for both mandatory and spontaneous breaths
- Peak inspiratory pressure, which will increase with increased airway resistance from secretions or ARDS

▧ Respiratory rate for both the ventilator and the patient
▧ Cuff pressure
▧ Appropriate alarms set and activated
▧ Pulse oximetry (SpO_2)
▧ End-tidal CO_2 ($PetCO_2$)
▧ Breath sounds
▧ Sputum
▧ ABG and lab results
▧ Hemodynamic values (if available)
▧ Patient comfort and tolerance of mechanical ventilation

TROUBLESHOOTING TIPS

All ventilator alarms must be on and functional to alert the nurse to changes in the patient's condition. In the event of an alarm situation that is not readily corrected, the nurse should use the bag-valve mask and manually bag the patient while another clinician troubleshoots the alarm. Common ventilator alarms are discussed in Table 3.2.

Clinical Pearl	It is important for the clinician to assess the patient for comfort and patient ventilator dyssynchrony, as the ABGs and SaO_2 may be within the normal range, yet the patient's work of breathing is increased. Fine tuning of the settings is necessary to make the patient comfortable and reduce the work of breathing.

FUTURE CONSIDERATIONS IN VENTILATOR SUPPORT

There is a paucity of research on the different ventilator modes to determine whether one is superior to the others. Current research has established that smaller V_T of 6 mL/kg of ideal body weight and limiting inspiratory plateau pressure to 30 cm H_2O have become best practice in the management of acute lung injury and ARDS (Haas & Bauser, 2012). Some ventilator modes are unique to the manufacturer and not all ventilators have the capability to achieve certain functions. Smart technology may improve the mechanics of the ventilator to automate processes such as weaning. A new innovation offering a lung-protective strategy is adaptive-support ventilation. With this technology, the target minute volume

Table 3.2 ▨ *Common Ventilator Alarms*

Alarm Condition	Cause	Nursing Intervention
High pressure	Will alarm if pressure increases in the circuit due to secretions, coughing, kinked tubing, water obstructing the tubing, patient biting the endotracheal tube, bronchospasm, lowered lung compliance, pneumothorax, right mainstem intubation	• Bite block to prevent patient from biting on tube • Auscultate for migration of tube into right mainstem bronchus • Administer bronchodilator for bronchospasm • Provide sedation as required • Drain water from the tubing • Chest x-ray to assess for pathological conditions such as pulmonary edema or ARDS • Assess for tension pneumothorax
High-exhaled volume	When the volumes of gas are larger than set levels	• Assess for change in patient condition, such as increased respiratory rate, and treat underlying cause • Assess for inappropriate ventilator settings such as too high V_T and correct the setting
Low-exhaled volume	Alarms with possible air leak	• Auscultate patient's neck area for evidence of possible leak around tube or displacement of the tube above the vocal cords • Assess patient circuit for possible leak or disconnection • Assess for leak in chest tube • Check for ventilator malfunction

(continued)

Table 3.2 ▨ *Common Ventilator Alarms* (*continued*)

Alarm Condition	Cause	Nursing Intervention
Low inspiratory pressure	Alarms when there is a leak in the system	• Determine cause of leak and correct • Assess for increased spontaneous breathing • Assess for displacement of the tube • Check for ventilator malfunction
Apnea	Alarms when no exhalation is detected for approximately 20 seconds	• Assess patient for cause of apnea and change mode • If patient is in an arrest situation, use bag-valve mask and manually bag patient while performing resuscitative measures
Low oxygen	Loss of pressure in the oxygen lines	• Check O_2 hose for accidental disconnect • Provide portable O_2 source and manually bag patient if main O_2 source is unstable
Low PEEP	PEEP is not being maintained	• Assess circuit for a leak
High exhaled tidal volume or high minute ventilation	High respiratory rate or increase in tidal volume	• Assess underlying cause of high respiratory rate such as pain, anxiety, hypoxemia, or metabolic acidosis • Drain any excess water in the tubing appropriately

Source: Grossbach (2008); Pierce (2007).

is set and the ventilator determines the appropriate V_T and rate based on the patient's respiratory mechanics (Hass & Bauser, 2012). Further research is warranted into the efficacy of new ventilator modes such as adaptive support ventilation. It is important to note that the clinician caring for the patient requiring sophisticated ventilation modes requires specialized education.

SUMMARY

Ventilator modes continue to evolve depending on innovative technology and ongoing research. The traditional modes of volume targeted ventilation such as assist/control or SIMV are useful when full support is required such as when the patient is emerging from anesthesia. The use of sedation and paralytics may be required to prevent patient-ventilator dyssynchrony. Pressure targeted ventilation modes such as pressure control is beneficial to the patient by permitting the patient to breathe spontaneously, therefore maintaining muscle strength and reducing deconditioning. Smaller V_T and limiting the inspiratory plateau pressure is consistent with best practices.

Questions to Consider

The answers are found beginning on page 133.
1. Compare and contrast pressure-targeted mode of ventilation with volume-targeted mode of ventilation.
2. What mode of ventilation is best for a patient emerging from anesthesia?
3. What collaborative care would benefit a patient experiencing patient–ventilator dyssynchrony?

Case Study

A 65-year-old man was admitted to the intensive care unit after experiencing an anterior myocardial infarction. He was at home working in his wood shop when he began having crushing chest pain, which he thought was indigestion from the previous night's dinner. He delayed calling emergency services for 10 hours. The pain was becoming bothersome, so he called emergency services. He has a history of a pack-per-day-smoker, diabetes, and hypertension. He was given morphine, nitroglycerine spray, and aspirin; and an ECG was obtained. Suddenly the patient becomes short of breath and has coarse crackles scattered throughout bilateral lung fields with pink frothy sputum suctioned orally. His SpO_2 dropped to 87%. The nurse changes the oxygen delivery system to rebreather mask with an FiO_2 at 1.0. His ABGs indicate respiratory acidosis with moderate hypoxemia.

1. What would be the most appropriate mode of ventilation for this patient?
2. What alarms would be important to set?
3. The patient continues to deteriorate and requires intubation and mechanical ventilation. What would be the most appropriate mode? In a collaborative approach, how would the nurse initiate mechanical ventilation?

REFERENCES

Bortolotto, S., & Makic, M. (2012). Understanding advanced modes of mechanical ventilation. *Critical Care Nursing Clinics, 24*(3), 443–456.

Burns, S. (2009). Critical care pulmonary management. In M. Wyckoff, D. Houghton, & C. LePage (Eds.), *Critical care: Concepts, role and practice for the acute care nurse practitioner* (pp. 49–88). New York, NY: Springer Publishing.

Grossbach, I. (2008). Mechanical ventilation. In M. Geiger-Bronsky & D. Wilson (Eds.), *Respiratory nursing: A core curriculum* (pp. 497–524). New York, NY: Springer Publishing.

Grossbach, I., Chlan, L., & Tracy, M. (2011). Overview of mechanical ventilator support and management of patient and ventilator related responses. *Critical Care Nurse, 31*(3), 30–44.

Haas, C., & Bauser, K. (2012). Advanced ventilator modes and techniques. *Critical Care Nurse Quarterly, 35*(1), 27–38. doi: 10.1097/CNQ.0b013e31823b2670

Kacmarek, R. (2011). The mechanical ventilator: Past, present and future. *Respiratory Care, 56*(8), 1170–1180. doi: 10.4187/respcare.01420

Kane, C., & York, N. (2012). Understanding the alphabet soup of mechanical ventilation. *Dimensions of Critical Care, 31*(4), 217–222. doi: 10.1097/DCC.0b012e318256e2fd

MacIntyre, N. (2011). Patient-ventilator interactions: Optimizing conventional ventilation modes. *Respiratory Care, 56*(1), 73–84.

Morton, P., & Fontaine, D. (2013). *Critical care nursing: A holistic approach* (10th ed.). Philadelphia, PA: Lippincott Williams & Wilkins.

Pierce, L. (2007). *Management of the mechanically ventilated patient* (2nd ed.). St. Louis, MO: Saunders Elsevier.

Pierce, L. (2013). Ventilatory assistance. In M. Sole, D. Klein, & M. Mosel (Eds.), *Introduction to critical care nursing* (pp. 170–219). St. Louis, MO: Elsevier.

Sole, M., Klein, D., & Moseley, M. (2013). *Introduction to critical care nursing* (6th ed.). St. Louis, MO: Elsevier.

4

Management at the Bedside

As many as half of all critically ill patients will require mechanical ventilation and specialized nursing care during their stay in the intensive care unit (ICU). Even though mechanical ventilation can be a life-saving intervention, there are many essential elements that must be monitored in patients receiving this treatment. Caring for patients who require mechanical ventilation is a core competency to acquire and develop for all registered nurses working in critical care areas.

This chapter provides a detailed approach to nursing care required at the bedside for monitoring a mechanically ventilated patient, including assessment, arterial blood gas (ABG) step-by-step analysis, hemodynamic monitoring related to mechanical ventilation, basic chest x-ray interpretation, and documentation requirements.

NURSING MANAGEMENT

Assessment

Well-developed assessment skills serve the critical care nurse well in detecting subtle changes in the patient's respiratory status. These foundational skills use the systematic approach of inspection, auscultation, and palpation to assist the critical care nurse in formulating an individualized plan of care for the patient.

History

The first step in a comprehensive respiratory assessment is to obtain the subjective data. Through a tailored approach, the nurse is able to obtain the necessary information without overtaxing the critically ill patient.

To acquire the necessary data, carefully formulated exercises and questions contribute to a thorough assessment.

1. Health history
   - History of frequent upper respiratory infections, allergies, asthma, bronchitis, chronic obstructive pulmonary disease (COPD), pneumonia, tuberculosis, or other conditions such as diabetes or cardiac disease
   - Past surgery, including postoperative ventilation or complications
   - Family history of respiratory illness such as asthma or emphysema
   - Medications prescribed or over-the-counter (OTC) medications, home oxygen therapy, or complementary therapy
   - Any allergies to medication, environment, or food
   - Environmental exposure in the form of occupation, animal exposure, recent travel, cigarette or cigar smoking
   - Calculate the pack-years history (number of packs per day x number of years smoked = pack-years) (Alspach, 2006)

2. Dyspnea
   - Have the patient describe any feelings of breathlessness or use a dyspnea scale
   - Ascertain exercise tolerance; how far can the patient walk without experiencing dyspnea?
   - Enquire about *orthopnea* or *paroxysmal nocturnal dyspnea*
   - Does emotion precipitate shortness of breath?

3. Cough
   - How long has the cough been occurring?
   - In what setting does the coughing occur; that is, cold weather, during allergy season, during exercise, related to medications such as angiotension-converting enzyme (ACE) inhibitors?

4. Sputum production
   - Note the color, quantity, odor, consistency, and the presence of blood

5. Chest pain
   - Use the PQRST (precipitating factors, quality of pain, region and radiation of pain, severity on a 1 to 10 scale, timing of symptoms) framework (Grossbach, 2008) to assess pain

■ Determine whether pain is related to the chest wall, diaphragm, or mediastinum as there are no sensory nerve fibers located in the lung

6. Miscellaneous
   ■ Body mass index
   ■ Enquire about other associated symptoms such as sinus pain, nasal discharge, hoarseness, weight loss, night sweats, or anxiety

Clinical Pearl	Use appropriate personal protective equipment (PPE) when performing assessment. Pay close attention to eye protection, as well as the mask (Weigand-McHale, 2011).

Note: In certain cases, the patient will not be able to answer some or all of the questions posed. Refer to the family or the patient's chart to ascertain the needed information, if necessary.

Physical Assessment

Following a systematic approach, much information can be obtained through the clinical exam using inspection, auscultation, and palpation. The skill of accurate percussion of the thorax is infrequently used, and is often replaced with other diagnostic aids such as a chest x-ray, computed tomography (CT), or magnetic resonance imaging (MRI) (Urden, Stacey, & Lough, 2010).

Inspection is the foundation of the respiratory assessment. A thorough inspection will mobilize emergency interventions if required, as well as yield important physiological data to formulate a plan of care. Alterations in level of consciousness and slight deviations in vital signs, especially the respiratory rate, will alert the practitioner to potential changes in patient stability (Massey & Meredith, 2011). First, conduct an overview or general survey taking particular note of the patient's color, level of consciousness, position in the bed, monitored vital signs, and ventilator or oxygen devices. In the initial general assessment, survey the environment for patient safety. Ensure all alarms on the monitor and ventilator are activated. Have equipment at the bedside such as a bag-valve mask and oropharyngeal airway in the event of an emergency (Lian, 2008).

Table 4.1 ▦ *Ventilatory Patterns*

Breathing Pattern	Description
Eupenia	Regular, even respirations, 12–20/min, approximately 500 to 800 mL tidal volume with each breath
Bradypnea	Abnormally slow rate of ventilation, usually less than 8/min; often seen with opiate overdose or increasing intracranial pressure
Tachynpea	Rapid rate of ventilation, usually greater than 20/min; can be a normal response to exercise, anxiety, or fever; also can signify impending respiratory insufficiency
Hyperpnea	Increased rate and depth of ventilation, resulting in increased tidal volume and minute ventilation; can occur in response to fear, anxiety, or exercise; occurs with metabolic acidosis
Biot's breathing	Irregular respiratory pattern characterized by two to three short breaths alternating with long, irregular periods of apnea, often caused by heart failure or renal failure; may been seen with increased intracranial pressure
Cheyne–Stokes respiration	Irregular respiratory pattern characterized by a rhythmic increase and decrease until a period of apnea occurs; carries a poor prognosis resulting in apnea and cardiac arrest

Adapted from Massey and Meredith (2010).

After the general survey, a close inspection of the thorax follows. Assessment of the respiratory rate, depth, and rhythm, including use of accessory muscles, will alert the practitioner to institute immediate interventions as required. Ventilatory effort should be observed in both the ventilated and nonventilated patients. Noting that signs of distress, such as central or peripheral cyanosis, tripod position, asymmetry of

Clinical Pearl Inspect the oral mucosa and lips for signs of cyanosis in patients with dark skin.

the chest, stridor, *paradoxical breathing pattern,* nasal flaring, splinting, and use of accessory muscles, require immediate attention and intervention. Observe the shape of the chest and the slope of the ribs. A normal chest will be elliptical shaped with ribs sloped at a 45-degree angle to the spine.

Following inspection of the thorax, auscultation of the anterior and posterior chest is completed. Expertise in listening to the chest will provide valuable data regarding the status of the lungs and pleural space. Auscultate for the presence of adventitious sounds that indicate an underlying pathology, such as congestive heart failure, atelectasis, or inflammation. When auscultating, compare side to side starting at the top of the thorax and move toward the lower chest. Listening in all three lobes of the right lung field and both lobes of the left lung field, as well as over the right and left bronchi and trachea, will ensure a thorough assessment.

The practitioner then palpates the chest to assess for any bulges, tenderness, or depressions in the chest wall. Assess for symmetrical chest expansion by placing open hands across the lower lateral aspect of the chest, with the thumbs meeting midline, making note of the chest wall

Clinical Pearl	For accurate auscultation place the stethoscope firmly and directly over the chest wall, never over a patient's gown.

during inspiration and expiration. Assess midline position of the trachea using the sternal notch as central reference, slip index finger to either side of trachea. Palpate, noting any areas of tenderness, instability of chest wall, or crepitus such as that found with subcutaneous emphysema.

MECHANICS OF BREATHING

Bedside pulmonary function tests provide information about the patient's pulmonary status. Data obtained from these tests assist in classifying the underlying condition, provide a baseline for the patient experiencing pulmonary disease, as well as for preoperative assessments (Alspach, 2006). The bedside tests are divided into two categories, each with four assessments. The most important tests for assessing adequacy of ventilation are reserve volume, tidal volume, and functional residual capacity (Diepenbrock, 2012). Other influences on ventilation are *compliance* and *resistance*. *Compliance* refers to the dispensability of pulmonary tissue. Conditions that decrease lung compliance, making it more difficult to inflate the lung, are acute respiratory distress syndrome (ARDS) or chest wall

Table 4.2 ■ *Assessment Abnormalities*

Abnormal Assessment Finding	Technique	Possible Cause	Intervention
Restlessness, alteration in mental status	Inspection	Early sign of hypoxia	• Administer oxygen • Determine underlying cause
Clubbing of fingers	Inspection	Late finding of chronic pulmonary disease or cardiac disease	• Supportive measures
Cyanosis central	Inspection	Arterial oxygen deficit	• Administer oxygen; determine underlying cause, such as low hemoglobin or decreased oxygenation of capillary blood
Peripheral		Low perfusion of the tissues	• Correct underlying cause, such as active warming measures, optimize cardiac output
Barrel chest	Inspection	COPD	• Supportive measures
Asymmetry of chest; one side larger than the other	Inspection	Tension pneumothorax	• Collaborative management: oxygen administration and lung re-expansion with needle aspiration
		Mucous plug	• Oxygen administration, suctioning
Inward movement of portion of chest on inspiration		Flail chest	• Optimize oxygenation with supplemental oxygen, chest tube and pain management

(*continued*)

Table 4.2 ▓ *Assessment Abnormalities* (continued)

Abnormal Assessment Finding	Technique	Possible Cause	Intervention
Tracheal deviation toward affected side	Palpation	Tension pneumothorax	• Collaborative management: oxygen administration and lung re-expansion with needle aspiration
		Atelectasis	• Reposition frequently, position with affected lung uppermost to promote re-expansion
Toward side opposite pathology		Pneumonectomy	• Position with unaffected lung in the uppermost position
		Inspiratory phase of a flail chest	• Supplemental oxygen/mechanical ventilation, pain management
		Neck tumors, thyroid enlargement, tension pneumothorax	• Supportive therapy
Breath sounds bronchial	Auscultation	If heard over the lung fields is suggestive of consolidation	• Chest physiotherapy, bronchodilator, expert consultation diuretic, oxygen
Adventitious		Crackles or wheeze	
• Diminished sounds		May occur in the bariatric patient, pneumothorax or obstruction within the bronchial tree, for example, from retained secretions or tumor	

deformities. *Resistance* is the measurement of the opposing force. Narrowing of the air passages due to a mucous plug will obstruct airflow, increasing resistance. Factors affecting resistance are categorized as patient-related or ventilator-related causes. Patient factors, such as bronchoconstriction, whereas ventilator factors, such as kinked ventilator tubing, will resist air flow (Pierce, 2007).

Physical Assessment

Care of patients requiring airway adjuncts is a key priority for nurses for both invasive and noninvasive airway management. Patients may have an endotracheal tube (ETT) placed to facilitate ventilation or a tight-fitting mask for short-term noninvasive ventilation.

▓ Assessment of the patient requiring noninvasive airway management begins with ensuring a tight-fitting mask to guarantee the correct tidal volume is being delivered. Protective skin dressings over potential areas of breakdown can prevent complications and create a tight seal. This tight-fitting mask can cause abrasions to the face, especially over the bridge of the nose. Take measures to prevent skin breakdown by beginning with assessment of the skin under the facemask every 1 to 2 hours. Avoid over-tightening the head and chin straps to maintain the tight seal, as this will increase patient discomfort.

▓ Invasive airway assessment or ETT management begins with assessing ETT placement. Common tube placement is approximately 21 cm to 23 cm using the teeth as the reference point. Securing the ETT is of prime importance to prevent accidental dislodgement of the tube. Various methods such as manufactured devices, twill tape, or adhesive tape can be used according to institutional policy. To prevent dislodging several tubes, secure each tube as a single unit. Maintain skin integrity around the lips, tongue, and oral cavity by repositioning the ETT. This may be done once every 24 hours just prior to the daily x-ray. The use of an ETT with a port to suction subglottic secretions will help prevent ventilator-acquired pneumonia.

▓ A tracheostomy tube is inserted to facilitate longer term ventilation. Assess size and type of tracheostomy tube and keep a spare in case of accidental decanulation. Special equipment such as an obturator should be kept at the bedside in case of accidental dislodgement. When assessing the tracheostomy tube, ensure that the ties are secured tight enough to allow one finger underneath to prevent dislodgement of the tube. Note any drainage on the dressing under the tracheostomy tube, as well as the condition of the skin around the tracheostomy.

Hemodynamic Assessment

Careful monitoring of the patient's hemodynamic status is essential, as mechanical ventilation can quickly compromise cardiac output and perfusion. When instituting mechanical ventilation, monitoring of all parameters related to circulation is required. Heart rate, blood pressure, pulmonary artery systolic pressure, pulmonary vascular resistance, and cardiac output can change depending on ventilator pressures. When documenting mechanical ventilation, make note of the relationship between the baseline vital signs and those after initiation of mechanical ventilation. Observe the trend of these values as there is no need to perform additional calculations due to the addition of positive end expiratory pressure (PEEP) (Pierce, 2007). Positive pressure ventilation causes increased intrathoracic pressures, impeding right ventricular preload. This results in decreased cardiac output and decreased blood pressure. The addition of PEEP further increases airway pressures reducing venous return. The influence of auto-PEEP may occur when there is obstruction to flow in patient conditions such as wheezing or in a patient with cardiopulmonary disease or with a high respiratory rate. A tension pneumothorax, a serious complication of mechanical ventilation, causes increased intrathoracic pressure. As a result, compression of the heart and adjacent blood vessels occurs, leading to cardiac decompensation and ultimately to cardiac arrest. Cardiac arrhythmias may result from hypoxemia during intubation or periods of suctioning (Grossbach, 2008). Suctioning may precipitate a vasovagal reaction resulting in profound bradycardia and hypotension. Always pre-oxygenate prior to suctioning, as well as observe the cardiac monitor during the procedure for tachycardia, bradycardia, or heart blocks (AACN, 2011). Aseptic technique must be used while suctioning. Alteration in renal function can occur in the mechanical-ventilation patient, as positive pressure ventilation can cause sodium and water retention, as well as fluid absorption from the humidification system. Frequently this leads to peripheral edema, pulmonary edema, and alterations in fluid and electrolytes (Alspach, 2006).

ROUTINE MONITORING AND CARE:
MECHANICAL VENTILATION

Listed below are routine requirements needed to ensure consistent monitoring of the mechanically ventilated patient. A number of these points are expanded on later in the chapter.

- Complete a comprehensive respiratory assessment, noting any changes in breath sounds
- Ensure that alarms are always on and audible
- Provide methods of communication (see communication section)
- Ensure stabilization of ETT and note measure at lip or nare
- Ensure head of bed is always elevated 30 to 45 degrees
- Reposition patient a minimum of every 2 hours
- Suction as needed
- Provide frequent mouth care
- Support the ETT so that it is not pulling on the patient's mouth or nose
- Anxiety, discomfort, and pain (sedation will be discussed further in Chapter 7)
- Monitor alarms (see below)
- Monitor any complications (see below)
- Hemodynamic monitoring (arterial lines, pulmonary artery catheters)
- Cardiac monitor and continuous vital-sign monitoring
- Continuous oxygen-saturation monitoring
- Assessing fluid balance and edema
- Eye care; prevention of corneal drying, injury, and ulceration
- Ensure adequate nutritional intake, dietary consult as needed
- Assess for subcutaneous emphysema
- Maintain muscle strength with active or passive range-of-motion (ROM) exercises every 1 to 2 hours
- Monitor trends in ABGs (see detailed section on ABGs)

**RESEARCH BOX: Manual Turns for
Mechanically Ventilated Patients**

The importance of manually turning patients who are unable to re-position themselves is generally accepted within the critical care nursing community. Despite this knowledge, it has been found that up to 90% of acute care patients do not receive the required manual turning and repositioning to prevent complications such as skin ulcers and decreased oxygenation. Winkelman and Chiang (2010) conducted a literature review of the studies that explored repositioning/turning of mechanically ventilated patients. Four clinical trials, two systematic reviews, and two meta-analyses were located that met the criteria. The findings showed that optimal turning schedule and positions have not yet been established and that additional research is needed in this area. It is clear that basic practices may not be followed in terms of repositioning mechanically ventilated patients. This is an opportunity for us to be vigilant and intentional in our manual turning interventions and follow up with documentation in order to improve the safety and quality of ongoing patient care.

COMFORT 101: CREATING A COMFORTABLE ENVIRONMENT FOR THE VENTILATED PATIENT

Tracy and Chan (2011) discuss a number of important nonpharmacological approaches that can be taken with critically ill ventilated patients to promote a comfortable environment. A summary of these comfort measures is listed below.

- Minimize noise, especially loud sudden noises, particularly during the night
- Access natural light to avoid the patient losing track of day/night cycles (avoid bright lights and harsh fluorescent lighting wherever possible, especially at nighttime)
- Relaxation techniques (i.e., progressive muscle relaxation, massage, especially hands, feet, shoulders)
- Communicate with patient and patient's family to determine patient's normal sleep patterns
- Provide music intervention (consider patient's preference, proper volume, and duration)
- Provide animal-assisted therapy (develop a policy on pet visitation)
- Imagery
- Promote a presence (physical, psychological, active listening, be attentive to the patient)
- Promote periods of uninterrupted sleep by clustering interventions and assessments together; sleep is essential in promoting healing
- Ensure comfortable positioning; smooth sheets and lift sheets

Table 4.3 ▦ *High-Pressure Alarms*

Potential Cause	Suggested Treatment
• Increased pulmonary secretions	• Assess lung sounds • Suction
• Patient biting ETT	• Bite block • Assess sedation level and sedate as appropriate
• Ventilator tubing kinked	• Ensure tubing is not kinked or caught in bedrail
• ETT cuff herniation	• Assess cuff pressure • Replace ETT
• Increased airway resistance (i.e., bronchospasm, coughing, pneumonia, ARDS, pneumothorax, pulmonary edema, atelectasis, worsening of underlying disease process)	• Treat underlying cause
• Patient/ventilator asynchrony	• Assess lung sounds • Assess for pain • Sedation • Positioning • Therapeutic communication
• Water in ventilator circuitry	• Drain water into reservoir provided
• Change in position that restricts wall movement	• Reposition • Keep head of bed elevated 30° to 45°

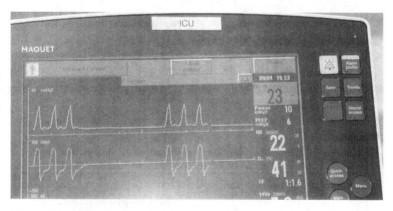

Figure 4.1 ▦ Ventilator with high-pressure alarm activated.

Table 4.4 ▨ *Low-Pressure Alarms*

Potential Cause	Suggested Treatment
• Patient becomes disconnected from machine	• Quickly reconnect patient to ventilator and ensure settings are accurate • Assess patient's breath sounds
• Leak in airway cuff • Hole or tear in airway cuff	• ETT will need to be replaced
• Insufficient air in cuff	• Assess level of air in cuff and adjust accordingly to create a seal
• Poor seal in ventilation circuitry connections (i.e., poor fit of water reservoir, dislodged temperature-sensing device, hole or tear in tubing, poor seal in ventilation circuit)	• Check all connections from patient to ventilator to ensure all tubing is connected and sealed correctly
• Loss of compressed air source	• Check function of compressed air source • Assess for ventilator malfunction
• Unintentional extubation	• Assess patient's breath sounds • Call for help • Manually ventilate with resuscitation bag as needed • Prepare to re-intubate as appropriate

VENTILATOR ALARMS

There are a multitude of alarms that may be activated while caring for a patient receiving mechanical ventilation. It is critical that alarms are always on while caring for patients to prevent life-threatening conditions from being missed. In order to provide safe, high-quality care to the critically ill patient, it is essential that causes of these alarms are diagnosed and treated in a timely manner. Some alarms on the

Table 4.5 ▨ *Patient Safety*

Patient Safety Alert: Alarms
• Ensure all alarms are on—always • Ensure ETT is stabilized and secured • Maintain inspired gas temperature at desired levels (between 35 and 37°C/95 and 98.6° F) to prevent thermal injury or poor humidity • Ensure suction equipment is at patient's bedside and is in working order

mechanical ventilator are activated by high pressure, whereas others are activated by low pressure. If the cause of the alarm is not quickly determined, the patient should be removed from the ventilator and ventilated with a manual resuscitation bag until the cause is discovered.

MONITORING FOR COMPLICATIONS

In addition to troubleshooting ventilator alarms, there are a number of additional complications of mechanical ventilation the critical care nurse must continually assess.

Table 4.6 ▨ *Complications and Interventions: Mechanical Ventilation*

Complication	*Suggested Intervention*
Unplanned extubation	• Call for assistance • Assess patient, breath sounds, respiratory effort • Patient may have to be reintubated • Assist spontaneous breaths if needed with manual resuscitation bag • Elevate head of bed to promote respirations • To prevent unplanned extubation: Administer appropriate levels of sedation, observe patient for restlessness, communicate with patient and explain all procedures (see communication section)
Gastric distress	• Administer antiemetics and medications to prevent gastric ulcers, as ordered (e.g., Ranitidine) • Insert a nasogastric tube attached to low intermittent suction
Complications of oxygen therapy/ hypoxemia	• Limit exposure to high concentrations of oxygen for prolonged periods of time as much as possible • Observe for signs of hypoxemia (decreased PO_2, decreased SaO_2, cyanosis, respiratory distress) • Observe for signs of oxygen toxicity (i.e., substernal chest pain, dry cough, restlessness, chest x-ray changes: atelectasis, patches of pneumonia, progressive ventilator difficulty)
Hypercapnia/ hypocapnia acid–base imbalances	• Monitor ABG results; observe for changes in pH, $PaCO_2$, HCO3, PaO_2. • Observe for signs of hypercapnia: hypotension, dysrhythmias, confusion, headache, flushed face, somnolence • Observe for signs of hypocapnia: tachycardia, dry mouth, palpitations, anxiety, profuse perspiration, paresthesia around mouth and extremities, dizziness, increased muscle irritability, twitching, seizures, coma

(continued)

Table 4.6 ▓ *Complications and Interventions: Mechanical Ventilation (continued)*

Complication	Suggested Intervention
Anxiety and distress	• Assess patient for adequate ventilator support • Communicate with patient (see communication section) • Assess patient for sedation level with an approved sedation scale and administer sedation as needed • Physician may consider neuromuscular blockade (see Chapter 7 for further discussion of sedation and pharmacological interventions)
Decreased cardiac output/ hypotension	• Monitor patient's hemodynamic status carefully observing for trends (i.e., PAP, wedge pressures, CVP, MAP, blood pressure [B/P], level of consciousness) • Monitor intake and output hourly • Patient may require fluid resuscitation and/or inotropic support
Increased intracranial pressure (ICP)	• Suction only as needed • Limit suctioning to less than 10 seconds and suction passes to two • Keep patient's head in neutral position • Keep head of bed elevated more than 30°
Ventilator associated pneumonia (VAP)	• Elevate the head of the bed to 45° angle when possible, otherwise attempt to maintain the head of the bed greater than 30° should be considered • Elevate for readiness for extubation daily • Use endotracheal tubes with subglottic secretion drainage • Initiate oral care and skin decontamination with chlorhexidine • Initiation of safe enteral nutrition within 24 to 48 hours of ICU admission (Safer Health Care Now retrieved from www.saferhealthcarenow.ca/en/interventions/vap/pages/default.aspx)
Pneumothorax/ tension pneumothorax (caused by volutrauma, barotrauma)	• Monitor for respiratory distress, pulmonary edema • Watch for fluctuations in B/P • Watch for tracheal deviation toward unaffected side • Watch for sudden changes and sustained increases in peak inspiratory pressure • If tension pneumothorax is suspected, disconnect patient from ventilator immediately, manually ventilate with a resuscitation bag, call for help, anticipate physician will insert chest tube and a stat portable chest x-ray order

(continued)

Table 4.6 ▦ *Complications and Interventions: Mechanical Ventilation* *(continued)*

Complication	Suggested Intervention
Sleep/rest disturbances	• Avoid bright lights, especially in the middle of the night • Avoid unnecessary noise or sudden loud sounds whenever possible • Cluster nursing interventions to allow rest periods
Patient/ventilator dysynchrony	• Communicate with patient • Ensure adequate ventilator support • Ensure optimal sedation levels • Provide a presence • Involve family members and significant others in support • Provide distraction techniques (e.g., music therapy; see communication section)
Aspiration	• Proper ETT cuff pressure • Elevate head of bed 30° to 45° • Provide antiemetics as needed • Set nasogastric tube to low intermittent suction • NPO
Arrhythmias	• Provide continuous cardiac monitoring
Vagal reactions postsuctioning	• Provide continuous cardiac monitoring • Limit duration of suctioning • Suction only as needed
ETT displacement	• Monitor and document placement of ETT • Order chest x-ray to confirm placement • Assess breath sounds every hour and as needed
Complications related to immobility clots, muscle atrophy	• Perform ROM activities every 1 to 2 hours (passive or active) • Provide early mobility wherever possible
Nutritional issues	• Assess nutritional status • Consult with dietician • Ensure patient is receiving optimal nutrition support early on
ETT occlusion	• Communicate with patient • Provide appropriate sedation • Use a bite block when necessary • Suction ETT as needed • Adequate patient hydration

(cotninued)

Table 4.6 ▨ *Complications and Interventions: Mechanical*
Ventilation (*continued*)

Complication	Suggested Intervention
Tracheal necrosis	• Ensure adequate ETT cuff pressure, ideally between 18 and 22 mmHg (Pierce, 2007); low enough to prevent tracheal damage but high enough to reduce risk of aspiration and pneumonia • Monitor cuff pressures by either *minimally occlusive technique* or *minimal leak technique*
Oral ulcers	• Frequent mouth care (i.e., with chlorhexidine swabs)
Ocular ulcers	• Keep patient's eyes moist with saline pads as needed to prevent corneal injury and potential ocular ulcers • Keep eye area clean and free of crust
Pressure ulcers	• Turn patient a minimum of every 2 hours • Observe for redness or skin breakdown, note particularly skin over pressure points • Provide a bed with special surfaces (e.g., air bed with rotating air flow) may be required, especially in longer term ventilation
Peripheral edema	• Monitor for dependent edema and hypervolemia • Monitor patient for need of diuretics • Carefully monitor intake and output
Subcutaneous emphysema	• Monitor presence and progression of subcutaneous emphysema • Document

COMMUNICATION

It can be very stressful for the patient to communicate with the health care team and family members when he or she is mechanically ventilated. While the ETT is in place the patient will not be able to verbalize because the ETT is inserted through the vocal cords; therefore, it is important to find alternative ways for the patient to communicate. There are six key steps to promoting effective communication with ventilated patients (Grossbach, Stranberg, & Chlan, 2011).

The first is to establish a communication-friendly environment. In order to do this, the nurse should reduce other extraneous noise as much as possible, face the patient while trying to be at eye level, ensure adequate lighting, and speak directly to the patient rather than from the side or from behind.

The second step is to assess functional skills that affect communication. Functional skills refers to vision (e.g., ensure the patient has his or her glasses on if needed), auditory (e.g., if the patient wears a hearing aid, ensure the batteries are charged and the hearing aid is working), and if the patient needs to hold a pencil to write a message ensure that the patient can adequately hold the pencil and has the strength to do so.

The third step in promoting communication with the ventilated patient is to anticipate the patient's needs in order to reduce anxiety around difficulty in communication.

Table 4.7 ▧ *Communication Assessment Tool*

Directions: Communication plan should be kept at the bedside and/or designated computer location so it is readily available to all health care team members and the patient's family. Update as needed.

Date assessed: _____ with patient _____ with family member_____ both_____

Mental status: alert, appropriate_____ lethargic, confused_____ comatose_____

Language:	**English:** Yes	No Other(List) _____	
Hearing:	**Normal**	**Impaired (R,L)**	**Hearing aid** Yes No
Vision:	**Normal**	**Impaired**	**Need glasses for reading:** Yes No
Writing:	**Right**	**Left**	
Grasps writing device:	**Yes**	**No**	**Unable due to hands: weak—swollen—**
paralyzed			
Literacy (reads, spells):	**Yes**	**No**	
Aphasia:	**Yes**	**No (If yes, consult speech therapy)**	
Neuromuscular weakness, paralysis:		**Yes (Explain)** _____ **No**	
Able to use standard call-light system		**Yes**	**No (Select adaptive system)**

Effective communication system(s) for this patient:

_____Nods head up, down to yes/no question

_____Clipboard, pad, pencil _____hand

_____Lip-read

_____Picture board

_____Letter board

_____Word board

_____Regular call-light system

_____Needs adaptive call-light system. Proper placement for use_____

Severe weakness, paralysis

_____Blinks eyes   1 blink = yes, 2 blinks = no

_____Moves eyes toward head for yes, closes eyes for no

_____Needs advanced system; speech consult sent

Details of effective communication system for Mr/Ms_____

Example:

12/6/08 Mr L communicated by nodding head to yes/no questions, needs glasses for reading and writes with right hand; elevate HOB at least 40°, points to picture board—usual issues have been pain, needs frequent position change, likes ROM to legs and wants radio on (AM 1500 or FM 100)

12/10 Update—same communication system as 12/6 except patient unable to write because hands swollen, weak, can't grasp. Discontinue pad, pencil for now

12/13 Bilateral hearing loss—MD notified, no ear wax—use Pocketalker in room

12/15 No change

HOB, head of bed; L, left; R, right; ROM, range-of-motion exercise.
Source: Grossbach, Stranberg, and Chlan (2011). Reprinted with permission.

Time				
Ventilator Parameters				
Ventilator				
Mode				
FiO$_2$				
V$_T$ (dialed)				
V$_E$ (dialed)				
Pressure Control				
Pressure Support				
PEEP				
Alarms				
Patient Parameters				
Patient rate				
Ventilator rate				
V$_T$ patient				
V$_T$ ventilator				
V$_E$ patient				
V$_E$ ventilator				
Peak inspiratory pressure				
O$_2$ saturation				
SBT				
ETT size				
ETT day #				
EVAC				

Figure 4.2 ▨ Example of ventilator flow sheet.

The fourth step would be to facilitate lip reading wherever possible. To enable this stand where the patient can see you (preferably at eye level close to the bedside) and ensure adequate lighting.

The fifth step is to consider using alternative and augmentative communication devices to facilitate communication when the patient is ventilated. Strategies can include having a clipboard with pencil and paper at the bedside, encouraging the patient to nod his or her head up or down or use his or her hand or facial gestures, writing down common needs (e.g., I am having pain) and having patient point to the appropriate one, and using voice sound boards.

The sixth step to consider in facilitating effective communication with the patient who is mechanically ventilated is to educate the patient, the patient's family, and the staff about various communication strategies and what the patient finds works best. By having a calm, confident, reassuring approach with the patient a more comfortable atmosphere will exist for the patient to communicate. Additional considerations include keeping the call bell within reach at all times, seeking assistance and strategies from colleagues, simple yes/no questions offered one at a time, and the involvement of family and significant others to alleviate anxiety and open up communication.

DOCUMENTATION

There are several important elements in documentating the ventilated patient. In addition to the patient's head-to-toe assessment findings, it is also essential to document the ventilator settings and the patient's response to these. Settings to document include the set tidal volume (Vt), the mode of ventilation, level of oxygen delivered (FiO_2), set rate, peak airway pressure, and adjuncts such as PEEP or pressure support. The patient's respiratory assessment findings, along with the oxygen saturation level (SaO_2), degree of backrest elevation, ETT placement, and any unexpected outcomes need to be documented as well. Each time mouth care or suction is provided to the patient, it should be recorded. Typically, hourly ventilator checks and documentation are performed in the critical care unit. In addition, any patient and family education should be documented.

DIAGNOSTICS

ABG Interpretation: A Step-by Step Approach

Monitoring the patient's ABG results is an important part of the routine of caring for a mechanically ventilated patient so as to determine the acid–base balance and level of oxygenation. There are four easy steps used to accomplish this interpretation and to be able to stay on top of changes in the patient's condition. First, consider normal values. The normal range for pH is 7.35 to 7.45. Values under 7.35 indicate acidity and values greater than 7.45 indicate alkalinity. The pH is an overall view of the patient's acid–base balance in the body.

For PCO_2, the normal value is 35 to 45 mmHg. Values over 45 are considered acidic and values under 35 are considered alkalotic. PCO_2 is primarily regulated by the respiratory system.

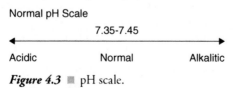

Figure 4.3 ▨ pH scale.

When analyzing bicarbonate (HCO3) levels, normal range is typically between 22 and 26 mmol/L. Values less than 22 indicate acidity and levels greater than 26 indicate alkalinity because bicarbonate is a base. HCO3 is largely regulated by the kidneys.

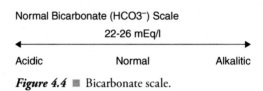

Figure 4.4 ■ Bicarbonate scale.

The level of oxygenation can be assessed by analyzing PO_2. Normal range is between 80 and 100 mmHg. Lower levels of PO_2 indicate hypoxemia. Typically levels of hypoxemia are classified as mild (70–80 mmHg), moderate (60–70 mmHg), and severe (< 60 mmHg).

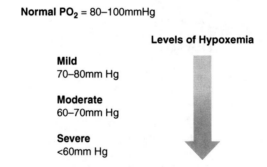

Figure 4.5 ■ PO_2 scale and levels of hypoxemia.

Step 1: Analyze the Numbers

For example, look at the pH, the PCO_2, the HCO3, and the PO_2. Is the pH normal, acidic, or alkalotic? In the example in Figure 4.6, the pH is acidic, the PCO_2 is high, the HCO3 is normal, and the PO_2 is low.

Step 2: Which Number Matches the pH?

Note that in Figure 4.6 the pH is acidic as is the PCO_2. Because they are both acidic, this indicates that it is a respiratory disturbance. Remember, the respiratory system regulates the PCO_2 and the

pH	7.32 (acidic)
PCO₂	48 mmHg (acidic)
HCO3	22 mEq/l (normal)
PO₂	78 mmHg (low)

Figure 4.6 ▦ ABG example: Respiratory acidosis with no compensation and mild hypoxemia.

kidneys (metabolic system) regulate the HCO3. Therefore, if the pH matches the PCO_2 the results can be analyzed as a respiratory problem (i.e., respiratory acidosis or respiratory alkalosis), whereas if the pH matches the HCO3, it is a metabolic disturbance (i.e., metabolic acidosis or metabolic alkalosis). In the event that both the PCO_2 and the HCO3 match the pH, this is considered a mixed acidosis or mixed alkalosis, meaning that both the respiratory and the metabolic systems are involved.

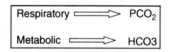

Figure 4.7 ▦ Respiratory or metabolic disturbance.

Step 3: Is There Compensation Present?

Once the nature of the disturbance is determined (e.g., respiratory acidosis), it is now important to determine whether the body is trying to compensate for this disturbance. If the patient is in respiratory acidosis, the kidneys may try to compensate by adding more base (HCO3); if this is the case, the HCO3 levels will rise above the normal range. If the patient is in a respiratory alkalosis, the kidneys may compensate by decreasing levels of bicarbonate and the results would be an HCO3 level lower than the normal range.

Conversely, if the patient is in a metabolic disturbance, the respiratory system "kicks in" to regulate the levels of acid (PCO_2 levels). For example, if the patient is in metabolic acidosis, the lungs may react by lowering the PCO_2 levels to compensate (in this case, the patient may be hyperventilating—"blowing off CO_2.").

There are three levels of compensation: full, partial, and none. In full compensation, the respiratory system compensates for the metabolic system or vice versa and the pH returns to normal. In partial compensation, the numbers begin to show improvement but the pH has not yet returned to normal. When there is no level of compensation the systems (metabolic for respiratory and vice versa) do not show compensation and the pH remains abnormal (see Figure 4.8).

Example 1: No (Absent) Compensation

pH	7.33 (acidic)
PCO₂	49 mmHg (acidic)
HCO3	23 mEq/l (normal)
PO₂	80 mmHg (normal)

Note in example 1: This is respiratory acidosis but the bicarbonate is not yet increasing to provide compensation there for compensation is absent in this case.

Example 2: Partial Compensation

pH	7.34 (acidic)
PCO₂	49 mmHg (acidic)
HCO3	28 mEq/l (high)
PO₂	80 mmHg (normal)

Note in example 2: The bicarbonate has increased to compensate for the respiratory acidosis but the pH has not yet normalized so there is only partial compensation.

Example 3: Full Compensation

pH	7.35(normal)
PCO₂	49 mmHg (acidic)
HCO3	29 mEq/l (high)
PO₂	80 mmHg (normal)

Note in example 3: The bicarbonate has increased enough to provide full compensation as evidenced by the fact the pH has returned to normal.

Figure 4.8 ▧ Levels of compensation: three examples.

Example 1: Hypoxemia

pH	7.31 (acidic)
PCO$_2$	55 mmHg (acidic)
HCO3	23 mEq/l (normal)
PO$_2$	62 mmHg (low)

Answer to example 1: This is an example of respiratory acidosis with no compensation and moderate hypoxemia.

Figure 4.9 ▨ Levels of hypoxemia: example.

Step 4: Level of Hypoxemia

In order to analyze the level of hypoxemia, the PO$_2$ levels must be assessed. Determine whether there is mild, moderate, or severe hypoxemia.

Putting It All Together

In order to complete the analysis, we must put all four steps together. See the practice examples and the accompanying full analysis below. Note that each ABG analyzed has three parts to interpretation: the disturbance, the compensation level, and the level of hypoxemia, if any.

CHEST X-RAY INTERPRETATION: THE BASICS

Chest X-Ray Interpretation

Most patients in the critical care area will require bedside radiography, such as a portable chest x-ray. When reading x-rays may be outside the scope of practice for the bedside nurse, a basic understanding of normal structures and correct line placement will be helpful when advocating for a timely intervention. First, a good-quality portable chest x-ray is taken by the technician using an anterior–posterior approach. To assist with this, the bedside nurse can place electrocardiogram leads out of the field of the x-ray beam. Other medical devices such as ventilator tubing or pulse generators may require repositioning as they can also obscure the view. Positioning of the patient in a high Fowler's position against the x-ray cassette with the x-ray tube at least 6 feet away will increase the clarity of the picture.

Example 1

pH	7.30 (acidic)
PCO$_2$	57 mmHg (acidic)
HCO3	25 mEq/l (normal)
PO$_2$	58 mmHg (low)

Answer example 1: This is an example of respiratory acidosis with no compensation and severe hypoxemia.

Example 2

pH	7.49 (acidic)
PCO$_2$	32 mmHg (alkalitic)
HCO3	29 mEq/l (normal)
PO$_2$	76 mmHg (low)

Answer example 1: This is an example of respiratory and metabolic (mixed) alkalosis with no compensation and mild hypoxemia.

Example 3

pH	7.48 (acidic)
PCO$_2$	47 mmHg (acidic)
HCO3	30 mEq/l (alkalotic)
PO$_2$	86 mmHg (low)

Answer example 1: This is an example of metabolic alkalosis with partial compensation and no hypoxemia.

Figure 4.10 ▨ ABG interpretation: three examples.

The developed x-ray film will vary from white to black depending on how easily the underlying structures are penetrated with the x-ray beam. Areas easily penetrated will appear black, whereas areas that are difficult to penetrate, such as pacemaker implants, will appear white, whereas structures such as the heart will appear gray (Ku, 2012).

Follow a systematic approach to chest x-ray interpretation (Ku, 2012):

1. Identify the patient using two identifiers. Ensure interpretation of correct film.
2. Identify view of x-ray to ensure the patient's left side is on the right side of the x-ray film.

3. Confirm the quality of the x-ray by visualizing vertebral bodies. If visible, the x-ray penetration is satisfactory.
4. Determine whether the patient is rotated by examining the symmetry of the medial end of the clavicle to the spinous process.
5. Confirm the trachea is in the midline position, which will appear as a gray shadow, with the mediastinum appearing whiter on the film.
6. Inspect the bony structures for symmetry. Identify nine to ten pairs of ribs seen posteriorly. Clavicle, ribs, scapulae, and spine are examined for any fractures. Assess interspaces for any widening.
7. Review the size and shape of the heart. The heart will fill 50% of the thorax.
8. Evaluate the diaphragm, including sharp costophrenic angles. The right hemi-diaphragm is 1 to 2 cm/0.78 to 1.56 inches higher than the left. A gastric stomach bubble may be visible.
9. Examine all lung and chest wall borders, as well as the subcutaneous tissues, for air or fluid accumulation. Look for any abnormalities in density for each of the lung fields, mediastinum, and surrounding tissues.
10. Identify tubes, lines, wires, and catheters that may be present. Compare current x-ray with previous films.

Table 4.8 ▥ *Tube Positions*

Device	Location
Endotracheal tube	3 to 5 cm/1.2 to 2 inches above the carina
Chest tubes	All openings inside the chest wall
Central line	Tip should be in superior vena cava, above right atrium
Pulmonary artery catheter	Tip should be in proximal right or left pulmonary artery about 2 cm/1 inch from the hilum
Intra-aortic balloon pump	Tip should be in descending aorta, distal to the left subclavian artery, approximately second to third intercostals space
Temporary transvenous pacemaker	Tip should be located in the apex of the right ventricle
Implantable cardioverter defibrillator	Lead should be in superior vena cava or brachiocephalic vein and the apex of right ventricle

Adapted from Ku (2012).

BEDSIDE MONITORING

Bedside monitoring devices such as pulse oximetry and capnography alert the practitioner to subtle changes in the patient's condition. Rapid interpretation with clinical findings will prompt early interventions.

■ Pulse oximetry is a way to monitor arterial oxygen saturation through a sensor placed on the finger, earlobe, bridge of the nose, or the forehead. The probe emits two light sources through the arterial vascular bed to a receptor on the other side of the probe. Pulse oximetry has a high degree of accuracy; however, in certain states, such as low-flow states, accuracy diminishes. Inaccurate findings may occur in low-perfusion states, motion, abnormal hemoglobin, intravascular dyes, exposure to light sources, and fingernail polish or nail enhancements,

■ Capnography is the measurement of CO_2 levels of expired gases with a monitoring device. End-tidal carbon dioxide ($PETCO_2$) monitoring is used for assessing effectiveness of mechanical ventilation, monitoring of CO_2 production, determining placement of the endotracheal tube, and establishing the relationship between arterial carbon dioxide and expired carbon dioxide. Arterial carbon dioxide is approximately 5 mmHg higher than expired carbon dioxide. Conditions that result in a decreased blood flow to the lungs (e.g., pulmonary emboli) will result in decreased $PETCO_2$. Increased $PETCO_2$ can occur in conditions that cause a decrease in minute ventilation, retained secretions, or increased production of CO_2 (e.g, seizures, fever; Grossbach, 2008).

> *Clinical Pearl*   Ensure accuracy of pulse oximetry by correlating palpated heart rate with monitored heart rate.

■ Calculating the PaO_2/FiO_2 ratio will provide a quick assessment of lung function. Values under 286 indicate worsening lung function.
■ Mixed venous blood sampling from a pulmonary artery catheter or via a fiber-optic catheter positioned in the superior vena cava afford valuable information regarding oxygenation. Mixed venous blood gases obtained from the pulmonary artery catheter (SvO_2) are slightly lower than the sample obtained from the fiber-optic catheter centrally placed in the superior vena cava ($ScvO_2$). Normal values for SvO_2 and $ScvO_2$ are 60% to 80%. This is altered when there is a

Table 4.9 ▨ *How to calculate the PaO$_2$/FiO$_2$*

PaO$_2$ ÷ FiO$_2$
$80 \div 0.21 = 380$
Intrapulmonary shunting is not occurring as the value is above 286.

decrease in oxygen delivery; for example, decrease in cardiac output, low hemoglobin, or an increase in oxygen demands.

▨ The arterial–alveolar gradient (A–a gradient) will assess for adequacy of oxygenation. This calculation represents the difference between the calculated alveolar oxygen and the measured arterial oxygen. This value is useful when determining the cause of hypoventilation. A normal value on room air is considered 10 to 15 mmHg, although it is influenced by age, supplemental oxygen, and barometric pressure.

Table 4.10 ▨ *Abnormalities of Mixed Venous Saturation*

Increased Mixed Venous Saturation	Decreased Mixed Venous Saturation
• Supplemental oxygen	• Hypoxemia
• Hypothermia	• Cardiogenic shock
• Sepsis	• Increased metabolic demands such
• Anesthesia	as shivering, seizures, hyperthermia, nursing interventions

From Urden, Stacey, and Lough (2010).

Table 4.11 ▨ *A–a Gradient Formula*

Aveolar	Arterial
$(FiO_2 \times 713) - PaCO_2 \div 0.8$	PaO$_2$ = 110 mmHg
⇩	
$(0.40 \times 713) - 35 \div 0.8$	
⇩	
$(285.2) - (43.75)$	
⇩	
$241 - 110 = 131$	

**Indicates pulmonary dysfunction.

From Diepenbrock (2012).

SUMMARY

The care of the patient requiring mechanical ventilation is complex and requires the critical care nurse to have a broad range of skills in order to safely care for these patients. This chapter discussed in detail:

- Routine nursing care of the patient requiring mechanical ventilation according to evidence-based guidelines
- Key priorities such as monitoring, assessments, complications of mechanical ventilation and suggested interventions, communication with the intubated patient, and documentation
- ABG analysis
- Basic chest x-ray interpretation

The scope of practice for the critical care nurse will vary from jurisdiction to jurisdiction. The critical care nurse must have knowledge of many elements of practice that may fall under the role of other members of the interprofessional team. It is prudent for the critical care nurse to follow institutional policy and regulatory guidelines when caring for the ventilated patient.

Questions to Consider

The answers are found beginning on page 133.

1. Analyze the following ABG result:

   pH   7.30
   PCO_2 30
   HCO3   20
   PO_2 72

2. What strategies would you consider to promote communication with a ventilated patient when using a clipboard and pencil?
3. Why must the head of the bed be elevated 30 to 45 degrees at all times when caring for a mechanically ventilated patient?
4. What are the potential causes of high pressure alarms?
5. List a minimum of five measures used to promote comfort in the ventilated patient.
6. A patient in the ICU has a centrally placed fiber-optic catheter to monitor the mixed venous oxygen saturation. The

ScvO$_2$ is 84% and is trending up. What is the nurse's analysis of this finding and the nursing priority?

7. The nurse is reviewing the chest x-ray and notes a large area that is radiolucent (black) on the patient's right lung field, there are no apparent vascular markings, lung margin is not in contact with the chest wall, and there is a mediastinal shift. What is occurring?

Case Study

Mr. Samuel Geldhart, 72 years old, was admitted to the critical care unit after a left pneumonectomy for cancer of the lung. He has a 25 pack-year history of smoking and has type 2 diabetes. His initial vital signs are stable. The patient is placed on a mechanical ventilator with the following settings: pressure control of 34, respiratory rate of 20 bpm, 5 cm of PEEP, and FiO$_2$ of 0.60. What are the critical care nurse's priority assessments? What is the nurse's first intervention?

REFERENCES

Alspach, J. (2006). *Core curriculum for critical care nursing* (6th ed.). Philadelphia, PA: Saunders Elsevier.

Diepenbrock, N. (2012). *Quick reference to critical care.* Philadelphia, PA: Lippincott Williams & Wilkins.

Geiger-Bronsky, M., & Wilson, D. (2008). *Respiratory nursing: A core curriculum.* New York, NY: Springer Publishing.

Grossbach, I. (2008). Mechanical ventilation. In M. Geiger-Bronsky & D. Wilson (Eds.), *Respiratory nursing: A core curriculum* (pp. 497–524). New York, NY: Springer Publishing.

Grossbach, I., Stranberg, S., & Chlan, L. (2011). Promoting effective communication for patients receiving mechanical ventilation. *Critical Care Nurse, 31*(3), 46–60. doi: 10.4037/ccn2010728

Ku, V. (2012). A fresh look at chest x rays. *Nursing 2012 Critical Care, 7*(6), 23–29.

Lian, J. (2008). Know the facts of mechanical ventilation. *Nursing 2008 Critical Care, 3*(5), 43–49.

Massey, D., & Meredith, T. (2010). Respiratory assessment 1: Why do it and how to do it. *British Journal of Cardiac Nursing, 5*(11), 537–643.

Massey, D., & Meredith, T. (2011). Respiratory assessment 2: More key skills to improve care. *British Journal of Cardiac Nursing, 6*(2), 63–68.

Morton, P., & Fontaine, D. (2009). *Critical care nursing: A holistic approach* (9th ed.). Philadelphia, PA: Lippincott Williams & Wilkins.

Pierce, L. (2007). *Management of the mechanically ventilated patient* (2nd ed.). St. Louis, MO: Saunders.

Tracy, M., & Chlan, L. (2011). Nonpharmacological interventions to manage common symptoms in patients receiving mechanical ventilation. *Critical Care Nurse, 31*(3), 19–28. doi: 10.4037/ccn2011653

Urden, L., Stacey, K., & Lough, M. (2010). *Critical care nursing: Diagnosis & treatment.* St. Louis, MO: Mosby Elsevier.

Weigand-McHale, D. (2011). *AACN procedure manual of critical care* (6th ed.). St. Louis, MO: Saunders.

Winkelman, C., & Chiang, L. (2010). Manual turns in patients receiving mechanical ventilation. *Critical Care Nurse, 30*(4), 36–44. doi: 10.4037/ccn2010106

5

Weaning

Mechanical ventilation is required for patients experiencing apnea, acute respiratory failure, hypoxemia, or hypercapnia. Once the underlying disease process has been resolved the patient will require discontinuation or weaning from the ventilator. This chapter describes the assessment required, as well as techniques and challenges in order to liberate the patient from the mechanical ventilator.

TECHNIQUES IN WEANING

Approaches to weaning vary depending on how quickly the underlying condition has been corrected, as well as the overall health status of the patient. In all instances, weaning begins as early as possible to prevent potential complications associated with mechanical ventilation (Chlan, Tracy, & Grossback, 2011; Pilbeam & Cairo, 2006). Involving the interprofessional team and following a standardized approach based on evidence-informed protocols will yield the greatest success in liberating the patient from the mechanical ventilator (Haas & Loik, 2012). Practitioner-initiated or nurse-driven protocols in collaboration with other health care members positively impact the weaning process (Pilbeam & Cairo, 2006). Including the patient and family in the weaning process will decrease anxiety and prepare the patient for the weaning experience (Burns, 2011).

The approach to weaning is determined by the length of time the patient has required mechanical ventilation. Patients requiring mechanical ventilation for 3 days or less would be considered short-term ventilation and those requiring mechanical ventilation for longer than 3 days are considered long-term ventilation. To successfully wean a patient from the mechanical ventilator, an individualized plan of care based on standardized protocols is required. In conjunction with the individualized care plan, consideration of the length of time the patient has required mechanical ventilation must be given. There is a strong correlation between the amount of sedation used and liberation from the ventilator (Burns, 2011).

ASSESSMENT

In preparation for weaning a patient from the mechanical ventilator, the interprofessional team is consulted to address any barriers to successfully weaning the patient. In addition, regimens to prevent ventilator-associated pneumonia, deep vein thrombosis, peptic ulcer disease, and other prophylaxis should be maintained. The underlying cause necessitating mechanical ventilation should be resolved. Parameters to consider prior to weaning are:

- Hemodynamic stability
  - Minimum inotropic support
  - Adequate cardiac output
  - Afebrile
  - Hematocrit greater than 25%
- Respiratory stability
  - Improved chest x-ray
  - PaO_2 greater than 60 mmHg with FiO_2 less than 0.5
  - PaO_2/FiO_2 greater than 150 to 200
  - Positive end expiratory pressure (PEEP) less than 5 to 8 cm H_2O
  - Vital capacity 10 to 15 mL/kg
  - Spontaneous tidal volume 5 mL/kg
  - Respiratory rate less than 30 breaths/min
  - Minute ventilation 5 to 10 L/min
  - Negative inspiratory pressure greater than –20 cm H_2O
  - Rapid shallow breathing index less than 105
- Metabolic factors stable
  - Electrolytes within normal range
  - ABGs (arterial blood gases) normalized
- Other
  - Adequate management of pain and anxiety
  - Patient is well rested

The tools to screen the patient for readiness criteria vary from hospital-based checklists to well-validated and reliable tools such as the Burns Wean Assessment Program (BWAP). The BWAP is used for those patients intubated longer than 72 hours (Figure 5.1) to determine the potential for weaning from the mechanical ventilator.

Patient Name _____   Patient History Number_____

Patient Weight _____ kg

I.   GENERAL ASSESSMENT

<table>
<tr><td colspan="3"></td><td></td><td></td></tr>
<tr><td>YES</td><td>NO</td><td>NOT
ASSESSED</td><td></td><td></td></tr>
<tr><td>__ __</td><td></td><td>__</td><td>1.</td><td>Hemodynamically stable? (pulse rate, cardiac output)</td></tr>
<tr><td>__ __</td><td></td><td>__</td><td>2.</td><td>Free from factors that increase or decrease metabolic rate
(seizures, temperature, sepsis, bacteremia, hypo/hyper thyroid)?</td></tr>
<tr><td>__ __</td><td></td><td>__</td><td>3.</td><td>Hematocrit > 25% (or baseline)?</td></tr>
<tr><td>__ __</td><td></td><td>__</td><td>4.</td><td>Systemically hydrated? (weight at or near baseline, balanced intake
 and output)?</td></tr>
<tr><td>__ __</td><td></td><td>__</td><td>5.</td><td>Nourished? (albumin > 2.5, parenteral/enteral feedings maximized)
If albumin is low and anasarca or third spacing is present, score
for hydration should be "no."</td></tr>
<tr><td>__ __</td><td></td><td>__</td><td>6.</td><td>Electrolytes within normal limits? (including Ca, Mg, PO_4).
* Correct Ca^{++} for albumin level.</td></tr>
<tr><td>__ __</td><td></td><td>__</td><td>7.</td><td>Pain controlled? (subjective determination)</td></tr>
<tr><td>__ __</td><td></td><td>__</td><td>8.</td><td>Adequate sleep/rest? (subjective determination)</td></tr>
<tr><td>__ __</td><td></td><td>__</td><td>9.</td><td>Appropriate level of anxiety and nervousness?
(subjective determination)</td></tr>
<tr><td>__ __</td><td></td><td>__</td><td>10.</td><td>Absence of bowel problems (diarrhea, constipation, ileus)?</td></tr>
<tr><td>__ __</td><td></td><td>__</td><td>11.</td><td>Improved general body strength/endurance? (i.e., out of bed in
chair, progressive activity program)?</td></tr>
<tr><td>__ __</td><td></td><td>__</td><td>12.</td><td>Chest x-ray improving or returned to baseline?</td></tr>
</table>

Figure 5.1 ▨ Burns Wean Assessment Program.

Ca, calcium; Mg, magnesium; PO_4, phosphate

Copyright Burns 1990 (Burns, Fisher, Tibble, Lewis, and Merrel, 2010)

(continued)

II.   RESPIRATORY ASSESSMENT

Gas Flow and Work of Breathing

YES	NO	NOT ASSESSED		
— —	—	13.	Eupneic respiratory rate and pattern (spontaneous RR < 25, without dyspnea, absence of accessory muscle use). * This is assessed off the ventilator while measuring #20-23.
— —	—	14.	Absence of adventitious breath sounds? (rhonchi, rales, wheezing)
— —	—	15.	Secretions thin and minimal?
— —	—	16.	Absence of neuromuscular disease/deformity?
— —	—	17.	Absence of abdominal distention/obesity/ascites?
— —	—	18.	Oral ETT > #7.5 or trach > #6.0

Airway Clearance

— —	—	19.	Cough and swallow reflexes adequate?

Strength

— —	—	20.	NIP < -20 (negative inspiratory pressure)
— —	—	21.	PEP > +30 (positive expiratory pressure)

Endurance

— —	—	22.	STV > 5 ml/kg (spontaneous tidal volume)?
— —	—	23.	VC > 10-15 ml/kg (vital capacity)?

ABGs

— —	—	24.	pH 7.30-7.45
— —	—	25.	$PaCO_2$~40 mm/hg (or baseline) with MV < 10 L/min (minute value) * This is evaluated while on ventilator.
— —	—	26.	PaO_2 > 60 on FiO_2 < 40%

Figure 5.1 ▦ Burns Wean Assessment Program.

Copyright Burns 1990 (Burns, Fisher, Tibble, Lewis, and Merrel, 2010)

Incorporating the use of the BWAP or other assessment tools will ensure that all weaning parameters are addressed and the potential for failure is mitigated.

METHOD

There are several weaning methods that are effective in liberating the patient from the ventilator, with no one method proving to be superior. These include synchronized intermittent mandatory ventilation (SIMV), pressure support (PS), T-piece, or continuous positive airway pressure (CPAP). Current research recommends the use of the spontaneous breathing trial (SBT) in which the patient can demonstrate the ability to breathe without assistance of the mechanical ventilator (ARDSnet, 2008; Haas & Loik, 2012; Morton & Fontaine, 2013; Pierce, 2013). When using the SBT method, the goal is to gradually improve the patient's respiratory muscle strength and endurance to support spontaneous breathing. When the patient is able to maintain spontaneous respiratory effort and is considered stable for 90 to 120 minutes, the patient has passed the SBT. Depending on many factors, such as the length of time the patient has required mechanical ventilation, underlying disease process, and comorbidities, this may be a lengthy process taking days to weeks to accomplish. Prior to initiating a weaning trial, the patient must pass the weaning screen test (see Table 5.1). The patient is said to have successfully completed the wean screen when he or she demonstrates hemodynamic stability, FiO_2 is less than 0.50, and the PEEP is less than 8 cm H_2O (Burns, 2011). Predetermined criteria regarding the length of the trial should be established by the interprofessional team. The following modes are most often selected for the SBT:

- PS provides inspiratory support to overcome the resistance of the endotracheal tube (ETT) and the ventilator circuit. To initiate weaning using this mode, the PS begins at a level that provides a normal respiratory rate and tidal volume. Gradually reduce the PS by 2 to 5 cm H_2O as the patient tolerates. Some protocols stipulate reduction of PS by 2 cm H_2O daily or twice daily.
- T-piece weaning is accomplished through the use of an adaptor attached to the ETT, which allows the patient to spontaneously breathe humidified oxygen. This circuit does not rely on the ventilator; therefore, there are no alarms such as apnea, respiratory rate, or tidal volume to alert the critical care nurse of a deteriorating patient condition (see Figure 5.2).

■ CPAP allows the patient to assume the work of breathing through the ventilator circuit with the addition of PEEP to maintain oxygenation. With this method, the ventilator alarms will alert the critical care nurse to situations such as apnea, high respiratory rate, or low tidal volumes.

Once the patient tolerates the SBT for 90 to 120 minutes, the patient is rested on the ventilator by adding additional PS or ventilator breaths to achieve a respiratory rate less than 20 breaths per minute. After a minimum of 2 hours rest, the weaning process may be repeated, gradually increasing the SBT until the patient is performing the majority of the work of breathing. The patient is closely assessed for signs of impending respiratory failure:

■ Respiratory rate greater than 35 breaths per minute or less than 8 breaths per minute
■ Labored respirations

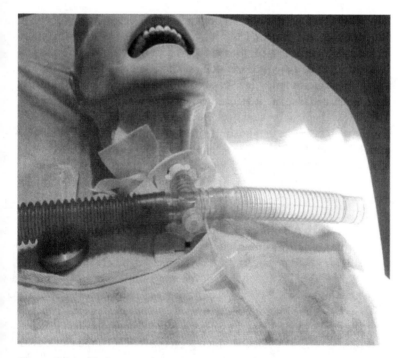

Figure 5.2 ■ T-piece weaning.

- Decreasing tidal volume below 250 to 300 mL
- Use of accessory muscles, for example, nasal flaring, intercostal, or substernal retraction
- Chest/abdominal asynchrony
- Oxygen saturation less than 90%
- Change in end-tidal carbon dioxide greater than 10%
- Heart rate (HR) and blood pressure (B/P) changes greater than 20% from baseline
- Diaphoresis
- Dysrhythmias
- Decrease in level of consciousness
- Agitation, restlessness, discomfort

It is important to terminate the weaning process at the first sign of respiratory distress to prevent respiratory muscle fatigue. The patient may need to have prolonged periods of rest (e.g., overnight) to recover from the SBT. The patient is considered to be successfully weaned when he or she does not need ventilator support for 24 hours.

Clinical Pearl	The critical care nurse is an important component of successfully weaning a patient from the mechanical ventilator. The nurse carefully monitors the patient, providing encouragement, and reassuring the patient that he or she can return to the mechanical ventilator as necessary. The critical care nurse should provide periods of rest during weaning and offer only necessary care during episodes of weaning.

Table 5.1 ▦ *Factors for Successful Weaning*

- Nutrition optimized
- Normal hemoglobin
- Electrolytes within normal limits
- Exercise tolerance through early mobilization
- Fluid balance optimized
- Pain management
- Psychological state
- Well rested
- Normalized glucose

EXTUBATION

Often used interchangeably is liberation from the ventilator with extubation and removing ETT. Depending on the length of time the patient is intubated, this process can occur concurrently. Especially for short-term ventilation, the patient may be extubated when assessment criteria are met (see section on Assessment at the beginning of this chapter). If the patient requires the mechanical ventilator for prolonged periods of time, a tracheostomy would be the most appropriate airway approach (Burns, 2009). The patient may then be liberated from the ventilator, and then decannulated once the patient is able to protect the airway (see Chapter 1 for tracheostomy management).

Extubation is considered when the patient is liberated from the ventilator and it is determined that the patient is capable of maintaining his or her own airway. If the patient has a strong gag and cough reflex and is able to clear secretions, a cuff-leak test is performed. This test is performed after suctioning the oropharynx, removing the air from the cuff, and briefly occluding the ETT. Absence of a leak around the cuff may indicate tracheal edema, which is treated with a short course of corticosteroids or racemic epinephrine prior to extubation. The patient is then extubated under close observation. If the patient develops stridor, racemic epinephrine via inhalation is administered.

Table 5.2 ■ *Steps to Extubation*

1. Assess respiratory status
2. Ensure that qualified personnel are available should reintubation be required
3. Discontinue feeding tubes 4 to 6 hours prior to extubation
4. Hyperoxygenate and suction ETT and the pharynx
5. Remove securing device or tapes
6. Deflate cuff and instruct the patient to take a deep breath
7. Remove the ETT at peak inspiration
8. Encourage patient to breathe deeply and cough
9. Apply supplemental oxygen
10. Monitor respiratory status, oxygen saturation, vital signs, presence of stridor or hoarseness, presence of larngospasm, and arterial blood gases
11. Be prepared to institute invasive or noninvasive ventilation

Source: Burns (2011); Pierce (2013); Pilbeam and Cairo (2006).

RESEARCH BRIEF

Research demonstrates poor compliance by critical care nurses to evidence-based weaning protocols. Often these protocols are complex and perceived as difficult to implement at the bedside (Burns, 2012). In order to integrate evidence-based practice, effective education strategies must be implemented for the health care team. To evaluate effectiveness of implementation of evidence-based protocols, an audit of compliancy and feedback to the team are required (Burns, 2012). Each institution should determine the best protocol to use in its intensive care units. Clinical judgment should supersede the protocol and not be replaced by a protocol (Pilbeam & Cairo, 2006). Expertise of the critical care nurse is vital to the weaning process.

Weaning protocols have been helpful in decreasing the number of days on a ventilator for patients with severe sepsis (Dellinger et al., 2013). Once the patient has met the criteria for the wean screen (arousable, hemodynamically stable, FiO_2 at levels that could be maintained by a face mask or nasal prongs, and minimal ventilator support), an SBT should be initiated. If the patient is successful, extubation should then be considered.

FAILURE TO WEAN

Despite meeting the readiness-to-wean indicators, some patients fail the SBT. Failure to wean is related to many factors, such as patient anxiety, premature weaning attempts, and sleep deprivation. Clinician experience plays a role in weaning the patient from the mechanical ventilator (Grossbach, 2008). If the patient fails the SBT, it is important to rest the patient overnight and attempt the SBT only once every 24 hours. Treating the reversible causes, such as pain, excessive sedation, fluid imbalance, and other organ dysfunction (e.g., myocardial ischemia), will improve the success of the SBT. To manage the care of a patient requiring mechanical ventilation, the critical care nurse requires educational support so that he or she is knowledgeable in evidence-based practice. A self-assured critical care nurse fosters trust and patient confidence, which in turn advances the weaning process. Having a consistent staff that can provide support and encouragement will also positively influence patient outcomes. Sometimes, however, a patient is unable to wean from the ventilator despite multiple attempts and will require placement in a long-term ventilation unit.

TERMINAL WEANING

At times, when a patient's condition is considered futile, withdrawing ventilator support is the most appropriate intervention. To initiate this process, a patient care conference is held with the interprofessional team, including family (and the patient, if requested) to discuss the patient's wishes. Once the patient's wishes are known, it may be necessary to consult the palliative care team to provide guidance and support for end-of-life care. It is important that the family understands that the patient may die as soon as the ventilator is withdrawn or the patient may not succumb for several days. Reassure the family that the patient will be made comfortable during this process with the use of sedation and analgesia. Dispel any notion that the medication will hasten the patient's death.

There are two primary methods of withdrawing mechanical ventilator support from the patient. One method is a gradual terminal weaning; the other is immediate withdrawal of ventilator support (Stacey, 2012). To begin the process, the room should be made comfortable for the family by dimming the lights, removing any unnecessary equipment, and by keeping the environment quiet and respectful. Remove unnecessary monitoring devices to avoid alarm situations. Discontinue any life-saving interventions such as intropes or other devices. To initiate terminal weaning, the ventilator rate is slowly turned down over a specified period of time in addition to reducing the FiO_2 to 0.21. It is important to provide analgesic and sedation, as well as bronchodilators to ensure patient comfort. The other method of withdrawing mechanical ventilation is immediate withdrawal by disconnecting the patient from the ventilator and extubating the patient. Immediately after extubation, the patient may exhibit transitory signs of respiratory distress, which are managed by repositioning the airway, and sedation. There is no research to support one method of terminal weaning over the other (Weigand & Williams, 2011).

In providing holistic care during this process, the critical care nurse should offer spiritual support to the patient and the family. Invite the patient's spiritual care provider to engage the patient and family in spiritually meaningful experiences at the bedside. As an alternative, after collaborating with the family, invite the institution's faith provider to attend to the patient's and family's spiritual needs. To illuminate meaning of this experience, encourage the family to recount stories about the life of the patient. Allow unrestricted access to the patient during this time. Removing barriers such as side rails and permitting unlimited visiting hours will foster an acceptance of the impending death. Encourage the family to touch and talk to the patient. Support for the family at this time is crucial. As death is imminent, prepare the family for the physical manifestations that may be encountered, such as changes to skin color, skin temperature, respiratory pattern, or reflexes. Respirations may become noisy as the lungs fill with fluid. Once death has occurred, the critical care nurse provides bereavement care based on the unique needs of the family. It may be necessary to provide a referral to counseling services for further bereavement support.

Providing end-of-life care is a stressful time for health care providers and may lead to compassion fatigue. It is important for the critical care nurse to arrange and participate in a formal debriefing with members of the interprofessional team soon after death occurs. This mutual support will assist the team members in providing quality end-of-life care.

SUMMARY

Liberating the patient from the mechanical ventilator should begin as early as possible. The first step in the process is to assess the patient using a hospital-specific screening tool or a reliable and valid tool such as the BWAP tool. Optimize conditions by ensuring that the patient is well rested, fluid status is addressed, cardiorespiratory stability is established, and oxygenation is within an acceptable range. An SBT is attempted once every 24 hours to maintain conditioning of respiratory muscles. Periods of rest alternating with prolongation of periods of spontaneous respiration are gradually increased. If the long-term ventilated patient is able to breathe spontaneously for 24 hours, then the patient may be extubated.

Questions to Consider

The answers are found beginning on page 133.
1. Compare and contrast short-term ventilation and long-term ventilation.
2. Describe the different weaning techniques and the advantages of each technique.
3. Provide a documentation note for the patient just extubated.

Case Study

Mr. Brian Snider, a 65-year-old male, underwent a double valve replacement 6 days ago as a result of endocarditis. He received two biosynthetic valves to replace his mitral and tricuspid valves. Past health includes a 45-pack-year history of cigarette smoking, mild chronic obstructive pulmonary disease, and hypertension. Mr. Snider required a prolonged period of time to stabilize due to postoperative bleeding. He returned to the operating room for exploration of his chest cavity for the source of bleeding. When Mr. Snider returned from the operating room, he required the use of intropes to stabilize his blood pressure. On postoperative day 5, the inotropes were successfully weaned. For the past 3 days Mr. Snider failed an SBT using PS 10 and CPAP 5 cm. Today, postoperative day 6, Mr. Snider successfully passed the SBT and returned to the ventilator to be rested.

1. What assessments would the critical care nurse make to determine whether the patient was ready for an SBT?
2. How would the critical care nurse advocate for Mr. Snider to facilitate successful weaning from the ventilator?
   On postoperative day 7, Mr. Snider was successfully weaned from the ventilator.
3. Describe the steps to extubate Mr. Snider?

REFERENCES

ARDSnet. (2008). ARDS clinical network mechanical ventilation protocol summary. Retrieved from http://www.ardsnet.org/system/files/6mlcardsmall_2008update_final_JULY2008.pdf

Burns, S. (2009). Critical care pulmonary management. In M. Wyckoff, D. Houghton, & C. LePage (Eds.), *Critical care: Concepts, role and practice for the acute care nurse practitioner* (pp. 49–88). New York, NY: Springer.

Burns, S. (2011). Weaning process. In K. Carlson (Ed.), *AACN advanced critical care nursing* (pp. 291–302). St Louis, MO: Elsevier.

Burns, S. (2012). Weaning from mechanical ventilation: Where we were then, and where we are now? In M. Mealer & S. Lareau (Eds.), *The lungs in a mechanical ventilator environment* (pp. 457–469). Philadelphia, PA: Saunders.

Burns, S., Fisher, C., Tibble, S., Lewis, R., & Merrel, P. (2010). Multifactor clinical score and outcomes of mechanical ventilation weaning trials: Burns wean assessment program. *American Journal of Critical Care, 19*(5), 431–442.

Chlan, L., Tracy, M., & Grossback, I. (2011). Achieving quality patient-ventilator management: Advancing evidence-based nursing care. *Critical Care Nurse, 31*(6), 46–50.

Dellinger, P., Levy, M., Rhodes, A., Annane, D., Gerlach, H., Opal, S., . . . Moreno, R. (2013). Surviving sepsis campaign: International guidelines for management of severe sepsis and septic shock: 2012. *Journal of Critical Care Medicine, 41*(2), 580–637. doi: 10.1097/CCM.0b013e31827e83af

Grossback, I. (2009). Mechanical ventilation. In M. Geiger-Bronksy & D. Wilson (Eds.), *Respiratory nursing: A core curriculum* (pp. 497–524). New York, NY: Springer.

Haas, C., & Loik, P. (2012). Ventilator discontinuation protocols. *Respiratory Care, 57*(10), 1649–1662.

Morton, P., & Fontaine, D. (2013). *Critical care nursing: A holistic approach* (10th ed.). Philadelphia, PA: Lippincott Williams & Wilkins.

Pierce, L. (2013). Ventilatory assistance. In M. Sole, D. Klein, & M. Moseley (Ed.), *Introduction to critical care nursing* (pp.170–219). St. Louis, MO: Elsevier.

Pilbeam, S., & Cairo, J. (2006). *Mechanical ventilation: Physiological and clinical applications.* Philadelphia, PA: Mosby.

Stacey, M. (2012). Withdrawl of life-sustaining treatment. *American Association of Critical Care Nurses, 22*(3), 14–23.

Weigand, D., & Williams, L. (2011). End of life care. In K. Carlson (Ed.), *AACN advanced critical care nursing* (pp. 1507–1525). St. Louis, MO: Elsevier.

6

Prolonged Mechanical Ventilation

Most patients requiring mechanical ventilation are successfully liberated from the ventilator once the underlying cause of the initial respiratory failure has been alleviated. For a variety of reasons, a small percentage—between 5% and 10%—of mechanically ventilated patients will require prolonged mechanical ventilation (MacIntyre & Branson, 2009). This small cohort of patients requires resource-intensive care, which accounts for nearly half of the critical care bed days and over half of the financial resources (Chen, Vannes, & Golestanian, 2011; Final Report, 2010). As more complex procedures are undertaken on higher risk patients, this trend is likely to continue.

To define prolonged mechanical ventilation, many clinicians have adopted the Centers for Medicare and Medicaid's (Department of Health and Human Services, 2011) description which states that prolonged ventilation describes the patient who requires mechanical ventilation for over 21 days. This patient may or may not have a tracheotomy. Conditions such as multi-organ failure, muscle deconditioning, sepsis, and delirium lead to ventilator dependence. Pre-existing conditions such as carcinoma, chronic obstructive lung disease, congestive heart failure, renal disease, and hyperglycemia contribute to prolonged mechanical ventilation. It is thought that if the patient is not weaned from the mechanical ventilator within 60 days, it is most likely this patient will become ventilator dependent (Nelson, Cox, Hope, & Carson, 2010). Patients requiring prolonged mechanical ventilation discharged from the critical care area have a high readmission rate, with up to 60% returning to an acute care hospital within the first year after discharge (Pilbeam & Cairo, 2006). Unfortunately, 55% to 77% of the patients requiring prolonged ventilation will die within the first year after the critical care admission.

QUALITY OF LIFE

Patients surviving the original illness yet unable to wean from the mechanical ventilator experience alteration in their quality of life

(MacIntyre & Branson, 2009). Simple activities of daily living become a challenge, with many of these patients having limitations such as difficulty with toileting, ambulating independently, and self-medication administration. This patient population experiences a greater rate of infection, delirium, pain, dyspnea, and anxiety (Nelson et al., 2010). These symptoms precipitate increased episodes of depression, contributing to a negative spiral.

Prolonged mechanical ventilation impacts the family, as well, as they struggle to provide emotional and physical care for the patient. The family is considered part of the team, yet often feels peripheral to any decision making. The family often is unprepared for the role of advocacy, which is required for their loved one. Aside from the emotional impact of prolonged mechanical ventilation, the family and the patient may experience a financial burden due to the prolonged illness. Loss of wages, in addition to increased costs associated with a chronic illness burden the patient's family (Nelson et al., 2010) as they struggle to maintain a normal life. The family caregiver often experiences burnout, especially in the postdischarge period.

Care of the Long-Term Patient

Care of the patient who needs prolonged mechanical ventilation requires expert nursing management. These patients face multiple challenges of debilitation, threats of infection, further respiratory compromise, cognitive deterioration, and enjoyment of life, as previously experienced. In working toward the goal of successful discontinuation of the ventilator, the team must be familiar with management of the mechanically ventilated patient in a post–acute care setting. It is often the nurse who assumes the role of the case manager. In this pivotal role the nurse facilitates effective communication among the team members, coordinating all aspects of care. The nurse collaborates with other team members to ensure integration of evidence-based practices, as well as compliance with the plan of care (MacIntyre & Branson, 2009). The frontline nurses are expected to adhere to policies and procedures, be knowledgeable in the management of a patient with prolonged mechanical ventilation, demonstrate effective communication with the team, and advocate for the patient. Nurses also need to be aware of the roles of other team members, such as the physician, respiratory therapist, dietitian, pharmacist, physiotherapist, occupational therapist, and social worker. Through collaboration of the interprofessional team, including the patient and family, goals are identified, creating plans to

Table 6.1 ▣ *Nursing Management of the Patient Requiring Prolonged Mechanical Ventilation*

Patient Goal/Intervention

Successfully weaning from the ventilator:
- Perform respiratory assessment/chest auscultation
- Use protocols to facilitate continued weaning
- Perform chest physiotherapy/ambulation
- Manage secretions
- Provide for periods of uninterrupted sleep

Nutrition:
- Consult with dietician
- Balance metabolic needs with nutritional intake
- Weigh patient weekly
- Monitor regular bowel elimination
- Monitor electrolytes and renal function as appropriate

Functional:
- Collaborate with physiotherapy and occupational therapy teams to strengthen the patient and improve conditioning
- Establish a daily routine with the patient
- Use splints and supports to keep extremities in a neutral position
- Encourage patient to meet basic needs as able
- Use tools to assess cognitive function
- Provide materials to facilitate communication, for example, note pads, calendar, pictures
- Encourage family to assist with simple tasks that are part of the care required, for example, range-of-motion activities, bathing

Prevent complications/promote safety:
- Ensure all alarms are activated on the monitoring system and ventilator
- Monitor skin integrity and take measures to prevent skin breakdown
- Monitor for signs of infection (e.g., pneumonia), remove any unnecessary devices such as Foley catheter, vascular access devices
- Strictly adhere to evidence-based practices, such as hand washing, meticulous oral care, and isolation techniques

From Morton and Fontaine (2013); Nelson, Cox, Hope, and Carson (2010).

successfully wean the patient from the ventilator, a slow process that could take months (MacIntyre & Branson, 2009).

DISCHARGE FROM THE CRITICAL CARE UNIT

Discharge options for patients who require prolonged mechanical ventilation are limited. The goal is to offer maximal rehabilitation as the patient is weaned from the ventilator. At times, the patient may not be fully liberated and will require lifelong ventilatory support. A collaborative, interprofessional team is essential to facilitate a cohesive plan with the patient. Each day, small steps must be taken to advance the patient along the clinical pathway.

In planning for discharge from the critical care unit, the interprofessional team must determine the best course of action. Early identification of patients who are at risk of prolonged mechanical ventilation is the key to the discharge process. The use of a screening tool, such as the Simplified Index Scoring Scheme, would assist in the early identification to move the patient along the continuum of care (Chen, Vannes, & Golestanian, 2011). This discharge process is complex as these patients often experience multi-organ dysfunction, thus requiring ventilator support in addition to other treatments, such as hemodialysis. Discharge options vary from region to region and impact the patient trajectory. The different models of care include acute care units such as a progressive care unit or step-down unit, a rehabilitation unit, a respiratory inpatient unit, free-standing respiratory care or home. Discharging the mechanically ventilated patient home is becoming more plausible as the technology evolves and support in the community improves (King, 2012).

Discharge from the critical care unit requires coordination of all services. The interprofessional team should include the registered nurse, physician, registered respiratory therapist, physical therapist, occupational therapist, spiritual or faith-based advisor, pharmacist, dietitian, social worker, discharge-planning coordinator, speech therapist, and the patient's family. Engaging in daily rounds provides a forum to discuss the patient's progression along the clinical pathway. A family conference begun early in the hospitalization and then held routinely with members of the interprofessional team facilitates open communication among all team members. This fosters trust and cooperation within the team to achieve the intended goal based on the patient's preferences. If the plan for discharge is for the patient to return home, early initiation of homecare agency services will allow ample time for education of the family and staff.

If the discharge plans are to a respiratory unit or an inpatient unit, such as a progressive care or step-down unit, the patient, family, and registered nurses need to prepare. Changes in the environment can create anxiety and mistrust for the patient and family. Easing the transition will be of benefit to all. Begin by decreasing the unnecessary critical care interventions such vital-sign monitoring. If the patient's condition is stable, monitor vital signs less frequently. Evaluate the need for the monitoring devices and remove them as early as possible. Introduce the patient to the new staff from the progressive care unit while he or she is still in the critical care unit. Providing an opportunity for the new staff from the progressive care unit to participate in the patient's care such as performing tracheostomy care, will facilitate continuity of care. This cultivates a relationship of trust between the patient and the nurses in the new area. A tour of the new unit with the family, and the patient if able, will decrease the anxiety associated with going to a new environment.

If the patient's wishes are to be discharged home, then the patient, the home environment, and the caregivers need to be prepared for this transition. The patient's physical status must be assessed and optimized for home care. Prior to discharge from the acute care setting, the patient's condition must be stable. This includes pulmonary status, ventilation settings, and secretions management. A home ventilator, referred to as an "assistive device" (King, 2012), requires patient and family education in order to safely manage this technology in the home environment. Multiple care providers should be educated on the equipment and care required for home management. Contingency plans should be established in the event of an emergency such as a power failure or deterioration of the patient's condition. Numbers to call in an emergency should be readily available to the caregivers. Appropriate signage to indicate that smoking is not permitted near the oxygen source should be visible. Assessment of the physical environment will yield information about electrical power and water supply, as well as heating and cooling in the home (Morton & Fontaine, 2013).

Transport of the Mechanically Ventilated Patient

Transferring a patient requiring a mechanical ventilator from one institution to another or from one unit to another can present challenges. Patient safety is the most important concern and guides the process in order to prevent complications associated with transport of the patient requiring mechanical ventilation. Advance planning is necessary to have the required equipment and staff available to provide safe patient transport. If the patient is stable, the respiratory therapist and the nurse should accompany the ventilated patient on routine transfers. If the patient is unstable, in addition to the nurse and respiratory therapist, the physician should also accompany the patient on transport. During the transport, the nurse should have the appropriate equipment to manage unexpected emergencies. Having access to resuscitation medications and a defibrillator will allow for early management of a patient's deteriorating condition. Communicate the patient's time of arrival with the receiving unit to minimize the time spent away from the unit. To streamline the transfer, minimize any of the equipment accompanying the patient. If possible, temporarily stop the enteral feeds and discontinue any intravenous solutions unnecessary during the transport. All lines and tubes should be well secured with adhesive tape or tube-securing devices to prevent them from becoming dislodged during the transfer. Finally, prepare the patient and family for the transfer to minimize anxiety the patient may experience with relocation from familiar surroundings.

All equipment should be able to run on battery power during the transport and have a spare battery in case of a delay arriving at the destination. The equipment should also have a low-battery alarm to alert the nurse when the battery power is low. To prevent acid–base disturbances, a transport ventilator is preferable to manual ventilation using the bag-valve mask (MacIntrye & Branson, 2009). All infusions should be administered using an infusion pump to provide uninterrupted flow. All alarms should be functional to alert the nurse of a hazardous situation.

When transferring the patient on a stretcher or in the patient's bed, the nurse should be positioned at the foot of the bed to observe the cardiac monitor and have an overview of the patient. The respiratory therapist should be positioned at the head of bed to ensure a patent airway is maintained at all times. Other personnel should be clear on their roles in a well-orchestrated transport.

Table 6.2 ▦ *Equipment Required for Patient Safety When Transporting*

- ECG monitor
- Blood pressure monitor (either noninvasive cuff or arterial line)
- Pulse oximetry
- Transport mechanical ventilator
- Portable suction apparatus with suction catheters
- Intravenous solution and tubing
- Defibrillator
- Emergency airway-management equipment
- Standard resuscitation medications
- Extra equipment such as spare trachestomy tube or chest-tube reservoir

Source: MacIntrye and Branson (2009).

Complications that may occur during transport include airway obstruction or accidental dislodgement of the trachestomy tube. Securing the trachestomy tube prior to transfer may prevent this complication from occurring. Other complications such as arrhythmias, hypotension, hypertension, and cardiac arrest may occur during transfer. With close surveillance, these complications are corrected with early intervention.

CHALLENGES

Managing patients with prolonged mechanical ventilation continues to challenge health care providers. Identified barriers include lack of early identification of patients at risk for prolonged mechanical ventilation (Chen, Vanness, & Golestanian, 2011; Final Report, 2010). There are few predictive screening tools to assist in early identification of at-risk patients. This patient population, although small, uses significant resources, which burden the health care system. These patients may be perceived as blocking beds or preventing admissions to the critical care unit due to their prolonged stay. To further complicate discharge of the mechanically ventilated patient to the home, the funding source comes from both the acute care and the community budgets. This can lead to confusion as to which pocket of funding is the most appropriate resource to use. Providing care for this complex patient population outside of the critical care unit is considered to be a low-frequency occurrence. Without critical care expertise, many teams may not be prepared with the appropriate skill set to provide the level of care these patients require. Strengthening post–acute care areas through nursing education allows for greater flexibility in the health care system. Finally, there are few data on this patient

---

Clinical Pearl To continue weaning the patient after discharge from the critical care unit, a goal should be established collaboratively by the interprofessional team, including the patient. Each day a small step toward the goal should be initiated. Incorporating a systematic approach using nurse-driven protocols will optimize the successful liberation from the ventilator or improve quality of life. If the patient cannot be liberated from the ventilator, a slower pace and individually tailored weaning plan are preferable.

population, which makes planning and funding difficult. By creating a central registry to improve communication among all stakeholders, the case management systems will facilitate the care needed for the prolonged management of the mechanically ventilated patient (Final Report, 2012).

SUMMARY

Patients requiring prolonged mechanical ventilation pose multiple challenges to health care providers. A collaborative team approach to weaning is necessary to move the patient along the continuum of care. Once the mechanically ventilated patient has been stabilized from the initial disease process, discharge plans should be initiated. When the patient is stable and ready for discharge from the critical care unit, there are a variety of settings the patient may transfer to, such as a progressive care unit or step-down unit, a respiratory unit, a long-term care unit, a free-standing respiratory unit, or to the home. To successfully transition to the postacute care unit, the patient and family need adequate preparation. Basic explanations and introductions to the new staff will alleviate some of the anxiety associated with discharge to another unit. To continue the rehabilitation process, the receiving unit has to adhere to evidence-based protocols. Protocols such as prevention of ventilator-acquired pneumonia will need to be instituted. If the patient is returning home, then the home may need to be modified to support prolonged mechanical ventilation. Collaboration across sectors is imperative to prevent further strain on available resources (Final Report, 2010).

Questions to Consider

The answers are found beginning on page 133.
1. As the registered nurse planning for Mrs. Mills's discharge, what options would be available to Mrs. Mills for discharge from critical care?
2. What would be the first steps in initiating discharge planning?
3. The nurse is transferring Mrs. Mills to the long-term care unit via stretcher. How would the nurse ensure a safe transport to the receiving unit?

Case Study

Daisy Mills, 72 years old, was admitted to the long-term unit in an acute care hospital due to failure to wean from the mechanical ventilator. Daisy was admitted to the critical care unit 10 weeks prior with respiratory failure secondary to right lower lobe pneumonia. Her chest x-ray has improved and the pneumonia has resolved. Past health includes cholecystectomy, hypertension, and chronic obstructive lung disease treated with home oxygen and bronchodilators. She has a 45-pack-year history of smoking. Daisy retired from the paint factory she worked at for over for 30 years. Her son and two granddaughters are waiting to visit her in her new room. She is experiencing dyspnea and anxiety as she settles into her new surroundings.

1. What are the key priorities in her care?
2. In order to advocate for Mrs. Mills, what are the first steps the nurse must engage in?

REFERENCES

Chen, Y., Vanness, D., & Golestanian, E. (2011). A simplified score for transfer of patients requiring mechanical ventilation to a long-term care hospital. *American Journal of Critical Care Nurses, 20*(6), 122–130. doi: 10.4037/ajcc2011775

Department of Health and Human Services. (2011). *Centers for Medicare and Medicaid Services (CMS) report: Determining medical necessity and appropriateness of care for Medicare long term care hospitals.* Retrieved from http://www.cms.gov/About-CMS/Legislative- Affairs/OfficeofLegislation/downloads/RTC-long-term-care-hospitals-final.pdf

Final Report. (2010). *Improving the experience of the patients requiring or at risk of long-term mechanical ventilation.* Canadian Institute of Health Research: Institute of Circulatory and Respiratory Health. Retrieved from http://www.stmichaels hospital.com/pdf/crich/sru-Mechanical-Ventilation-report.pdf

King, A. (2012). Long-term home mechanical ventilation in the United States. *Respiratory Care, 57*(6), 921–930. doi: 10.4187/respcare.01741

MacIntyre, N., & Branson, R. (2009). *Mechanical ventilation* (2nd ed.). St. Louis, MO: Saunders Elsevier.

Morton, P., & Fontaine, D. (2013). *Critical care nursing: A holistic approach* (10th ed.). Philadelphia, PA: Lippincott Williams & Wilkins.

Nelson, J., Cox, C., Hope, A., & Carson, S. (2010). Chronic critical illness. *American Journal of Respiratory and Critical Care Medicine, 182*, 446–453. doi: 10.1164/rccm.201002-0210CI

Pilbeam, S., & Cairo, J. (2006). *Mechanical ventilation: Physiological and clinical applications.* Philadelphia, PA: Mosby.

7

Pharmacology

PAIN, AGITATION, AND DELIRIUM MANAGEMENT

Management of pain, agitation, and delirium (PAD) in critically ill patients has greatly evolved in the past 10 to 15 years based on available literature and new evidence informing these practices. In this chapter, the most current guidelines in this area are highlighted and framed within a practical approach for bedside nurses caring for patients receiving mechanical ventilation (Barr, Fraser, Puntillo, et al., 2013).

Pain

Pain and procedural pain are common and not well treated in the intensive care unit (ICU). In fact, pain is 50% higher in both medical and surgical ICU patients (Barr et al., 2013). There are short- and long-term consequences to unrelieved pain in the ICU, which include insufficient sleep, traumatic memories of ICU, posttraumatic stress disorder (PTSD), hyperglycemia, impaired wound healing, and increased risk of infection (Barr et al., 2013)

Key recommendations for pain management include an "analgesic-first" approach and aiming for a target of lighter sedation in which the patient is able to self-report pain and to grade the severity of that pain, such as a 0-to-10-scale approach (Barr et al., 2013). Patients need to be awake enough to report their pain. For those patients who are unable to report pain, reliable and valid scales such as the Behavioral Pain Scale (BPS) (see Table 7.1) and the Critical Care Pain Observation Tool (CPOT) can be used (Gelinas, Fillion, & Puntillo, 2006). Vital signs should not be used as the singular method of assessing pain but may be used as additional information to assess pain.

In the analgesic-first approach, IV opioids are recommended for critical care patients with non-neuropathic pain (Barr et al., 2013). The choice

Table 7.1 ▓ *Behavioral Pain Scale (BPS)*

Item	Description	Score
Facial expression	Relaxed	1
	Partially tightened (e.g., brow lowering)	2
	Fullly tightened (e.g., eyelid closing)	3
	Grimacing	4
Upper limb movements	No movement	1
	Partially bent	2
	Fully bent with finger flexion	3
	Permanently retracted	4
Compliance with mechanical ventilation	Tolerating movement	1
	Coughing but tolerating ventilation most of the time	2
	Fighting ventilator	3
	Unable to control ventilation	4

BPS score ranges from 3 (no pain) to 12 (maximum pain).
Reprinted by permission of the Pain Task Force, Detroit Medical Center (2004).

of a medication will be individualized to the patient's situation based on such factors as the patient's hemodynamic stability, renal function, and onset and duration of pain. In addition to routine and consistent administration of these drugs for pain, they should also be considered preemptively in advance of painful procedures (e.g., repositioning, chest-tube insertion and removal). IV is the most common route of administration for pain medication because decreased gastrointestinal (GI) motility may be an issue. Adjuncts such as anesthetics (e.g., bupivacaine), acetaminophen, and nonsteroidal anti-inflammatory drugs (NSAIDs) may also be used to support pain control in addition to opioids such as morphine. There is not enough research evidence to support the sole use of these therapies in management of pain in the ICU. Thoracic epidural analgesia is recommended for postoperative analgesia in patients who have undergone an aortic aneurysm repair (AAA; Barr et al., 2013).

The most common pain medications in the ICU are morphine, hydromorphone, and fentanyl. See Table 7.2 for indications and important dosing and administration implications.

Neuropathic pain is not well treated with opioids and medications such as gabapentin may be used if administration via GI route is viable. Demerol is not recommended because of neurotoxicity.

In addition to pharmacologic management, it is important for the critical care nurse to also consider nonpharmacological interventions

Table 7.2 ▦ *Critical Care Pain Medications*

Medication	Route/Equianalgesic Dosage IV	PO	Onset (IV)	Adverse Effects and Notes
Morphine	10	30	5–10 minutes	Respiratory depression, bradycardia, thrombocytopenia
Hydromorphone	1.5	7.5	5–15 minutes	Respiratory depression, bradycardia, bronchospasm
Fentanyl	0.1	N/A	1–2 minutes	Arrhythmias, pulmonary embolism, deep vein thrombosis, respiratory depression

From Barr et al. (2013); Karch (2013).

to relive the pain experience such as music therapy and animal-assisted therapy. Furthermore, optimizing the environment by controlling noise and light, clustering care, and decreasing stimuli during night cycles is an important element in decreasing the patient's pain experience.

Agitation

In addition to pain, management of agitation in critically ill patients is a foundational skill required of nurses working in critical care settings. It is common for patients receiving mechanical ventilation to experience discomfort and anxiety leading to agitation in the ICU. In order to assess the level of agitation and promote comfort for the patient, the nurse must use reliable and valid tools such as the Richmond Agitation–Sedation Scale (RASS) and the Sedation–Agitation Scale (SAS) to monitor the level of sedation/agitation in the mechanically ventilated patient (see Table 7.3). The RASS and the SAS have been shown to have the highest psychometric scores on interrater reliability, convergent, and discriminant validation (Barr et al., 2013). Objective measures of brain function (e.g., auditory evoked potentials [AEPs], bispectral index [BIS]) are not recommended as a primary method of monitoring sedation levels.

There are many causes of agitation and anxiety among ICU patients (e.g., pain, delirium, hypoxia, hypoglycemia, hypotension, and withdrawal from drugs or alcohol) and it is important for the underlying cause to be identified and treated prior to administering sedatives.

Table 7.3 ▥ *Sedation–Agitation Scale (SAS)*

Level	Description	Explanation
1	Unarousable	Minimal to no response to noxious stimuli
2	Very Sedated	Arouses to physical stimuli; doesn't communicate or follow commands; may move spontaneously
3	Sedated	Difficult to arouse; awakens to verbal stimuli or gentle shaking, but drifts off again; follows simple commands
4	Calm/Cooperative	Calm, awakens easily, follows commands
5	Agitated	Anxious or mildly agitated; attempts to sit up; calms with verbal instructions
6	Very Agitated	Doesn't calm despite frequent verbal reminding of limits; requires physical restraints; bites endotracheal tube (ETT)
7	Dangerous Agitation	Pulling at ETT; tries to remove catheters, climb over bedrail, strike at staff, and/or thrashing side to side

From Fraser and Riker (2001).

Sedation doses can be adjusted or titrated to achieve lighter or deeper sedation levels; it is recommended that lighter sedation levels be used in the ICU. Improved patient outcomes are not only related to lighter sedation levels but also to minimal sedative use, the use of nonbenzodiazepines, and the use of reliable sedation scales and protocols (Barr et al., 2013). These guidelines have been shown to reduce the duration of mechanical ventilation, length of ICU and hospital stay, and decrease the incidence of delirium. Daily sedation interruption allows the critical care nurse to evaluate sedation level, downwardly titrate infusion rates, prevent oversedation and assess central nervous system function and recovery, as well as readiness to extubate (Concepcion, 2013).

Benzodiazepines

Of the three most commonly used benzodiazepines, lorazepam is the most potent followed by midazolam and then diazepam. Increasing age and liver and renal insufficiency can all contribute to delayed levels of sedation, prolonging emergence. Side effects of benzodiazepines include hypotension, respiratory depression, and cardiopulmonary depression especially when combined with opiates. ICU patients can also develop a tolerance to benzodiazepines. In addition, acute kidney injury and metabolic acidosis can occur with the administration of the parenteral form of lorazepam due to the presence of propylene glycol, which is in the diluent.

Propofol

Propofol is an IV sedative that has no analgesic properties; has sedative, hypnotic, amnesic, anxiolytic, antiemetic, and anticonvulsant properties. Because propofol has rapid onset and offset properties, this makes it an ideal medication for patients requiring frequent awakenings to assess neurologic status. Propofol is well suited to protocols involving daily sedation interruption. Long-term administration of propofol is not recommended because it can lead to prolonged emergence due to saturation of the peripheral tissues. Adverse effects of propofol include respiratory depression, systemic vasodilation, hypotension, bradycardia, hypertriglyceridemia, acute pancreatitis, and myoclonus (Karch, 2013). Critical care nurses need to be aware of the policy and scope of practice for administration of drugs such as propofol and dexmedetomidine as these drugs are typically administered and titrated by a physician. The critical care nurse has an integral role in monitoring patients receiving sedation.

Dexmedetomidine

Dexmedetomidine has a different pattern of sedation than propofol and benzodiazepines. Patients receiving this medication are more easily rousable and have less respiratory depression. Specifically in contrast to propofol, it does not have anticonvulsant properties. The onset of this drug is 15 minutes with peak sedation occurring at 1 hour. This drug has been approved only for short-term sedation (i.e., less than 24 hours) in ICU patients (Barr et al., 2013). The main adverse effects of dexmedetomidine include bradycardia and hypotension. It is essential that the nurse in the ICU continuously monitor respiratory status and oxygenation levels in patients receiving this medication as it can lead to airway obstruction in nonintubated patients.

Delirium

Delirium is very common in ICU patients and affects 80% of mechanically ventilated patients. "Delirium is a syndrome characterized by the acute onset of cerebral dysfunction with a change in mental status, inattention and either disorganized thinking or an altered level of consciousness" (Barr et al., 2013, p. 282). Delirium is associated with and a predictor of negative patient outcomes, which include increased hospital stay, increased mortality, and long-term cognitive impairment.

Key Points: Sedation in ICU Patients

- Underlying causes of agitation should be identified and treated prior to using sedatives.
- Nonbenzodiazepines sedatives (e.g., propofol or dexmetomidine) are recommended instead of benzodiazepines (e.g., midazolam and lorazepam) to improve outcomes in patients who are mechanically ventilated.
- Benzodiazepine sedation is associated with increased ICU length of stay.
- Objective measures of brain function (e.g., Bispectral Index [BIS], Auditory Evoked Potentials [AEP]) are not recommended as the primary method to monitor depth of sedation.
- Reliable and valid scales such as the RASS and SAS are recommended to monitor depth of sedation in adult ICU patients.

From Barr et al. (2013).

An important role of the critical care nurse is to recognize the signs and symptoms of delirium and to have an understanding of the assessment, treatment, and monitoring required. Timeliness in treatment of delirium is critical in order to reduce severity and duration. Prevention strategies include early mobilization and pharmacologic/nonpharmacologic interventions. No prospective research has verified the safety and efficacy of using haloperidol to treat delirium in adult ICU patients; further research is needed to study the use of any antipsychotics for this purpose (Barr et al., 2013).

ABCDE Bundle

Awakening
Breathing trial coordination
Choice of sedative
Delirium detection
Early progressive mobility and exercise

Reliable and valid instruments such as the Confusion Assessment Method for the ICU (CAM-ICU; Figure 7.1) and the Intensive Care Delirium Screening Checklist (ICDSC; Figure 7.2) have been shown to be the most sensitive in detecting delirium (Barr et al., 2013). In addition to implementing a delirium screening checklist, the use of the "ABCDE Bundle" for the ICU is recommended to allow for reduction of modifiable risk factors in delirium.

FEATURES AND DESCRIPTIONS	ABSENT	PRESENT
I. Acute onset or fluctuating course*		
A. Is there evidence of an acute change in mental status from the baseline? B. Or, did the (abnormal) behavior fluctuate during the past 24 hours, that is, tend to come and go or increase and decrease in severity as evidenced by fluctuations on the Richmond Agitation Sedation Scale (RASS) or the Glasgow Coma Scale?		
II. Inattention†		
Did the patient have difficulty focusing attention as evidenced by a score of less than 8 correct answers on either the visual or auditory components of the Attention Screening Examination (ASE)?		
III. Disorganized thinking		
Is there evidence of disorganized or incoherent thinking as evidenced by incorrect answers to three or more of the 4 questions and inability to follow the commands? Questions 1. Will a stone float on water? 2. Are there fish in the sea? 3. Does 1 pound weigh more than 2 pounds? 4. Can you use a hammer to pound a nail? Commands 1. Are you having unclear thinking? 2. Hold up this many fingers. (Examiner holds 2 fingers in front of the patient.) 3. Now do the same thing with the other hand (without holding the 2 fingers in front of the patient). (If the patient is already extubated from the ventilator, determine whether the patient's thinking is disorganized or incoherent, such as rambling or irrelevant conversation, unclear or illogical flow of ideas, or unpredictable switching from subject to subject.)		
IV. Altered level of consciousness		
Is the patient's level of consciousness anything other than alert, such as being vigilant or lethargic or in a stupor or coma? **ALERT:** spontaneously fully aware of environment and interacts appropriately **VIGILANT:** hyperalert **LETHARGIC:** drowsy but easily aroused, unaware of some elements in the environment or not spontaneously interacting with the interviewer; becomes fully aware and appropriately interactive when prodded minimally **STUPOR:** difficult to arouse, unaware of some or all elements in the environment or not spontaneously interacting with the interviewer; becomes incompletely aware when prodded strongly; can be aroused only by vigorous and repeated stimuli and as soon as the stimulus ceases, stuporous subject lapses back into unresponsive state **COMA:** unarousable, unaware of all elements in the environment with no spontaneous interaction or awareness of the interviewer so that the interview is impossible even with maximal prodding		
Overall CAM-ICU Assessment (Features 1 and 2 and either Feature 3 or 4):	Yes____	No____

* The scores included in the 10-point RASS range from a high of 4 (combative) to a low of –5 (deeply comatose and unresponsive). Under the RASS system, patients who were spontaneously alert, calm, and not agitated were scored at 0 (neutral zone). Anxious or agitated patients received a range of scores depending on their level of anxiety: 1 for anxious, 2 for agitated (fighting ventilator), 3 for very agitated (pulling on or removing catheters), or 4 for combative -1 for more than 10 seconds, -2 for less than 10 seconds, and –3 for eye opening but no eye contact. If physical stimulation was required, then the patients were scores as either –4 for eye opening or movement with physical or painful stimulation or –5 for no response to physical or painful stimulation. The RASS has excellent interrater reliability and intraclass correlation coefficients of 0.95 and 0.97, respectively, and has been validated against visual analog scale and geropsychiatric diagnoses in 2 ICU studies.

† In completing the visual ASE, the patients were shown 5 simple pictures (previously published) at 3-second intervals and asked to remember them. They were then immediately shown 10 subsequent pictures and asked to nod "yes" or "no" to indicate whether they had or had not just seen each of the pictures. Since 5 pictures had been shown to them already, for which the correct response was to nod "yes," and 5 others were new, for which the correct response was to nod "no," patients scored perfectly if they achieved 10 correct responses. Scoring accounted for either errors of omission (indicating "no" for a previously shown picture) or for errors of commission (indicating "yes" for a picture not previously shown). In completing the auditory ASE, patients were asked to squeeze the rater's hand whenever they heard the letter A during the recitation of a series of 10 letters. The rater then read 10 letters from the following list in a normal tone at a rate of 1 letter per second: S, A, H, E, V, A, A, R, A, T. A scoring method similar to that of the visual ASE was used for the auditory ASE testing.

Figure 7.1 ■ Confusion of Assessment Method for the Intensive Care Unit (CAM-ICU) scale.

Source: Adapted with permission from Ely, Inouye, Bernard, et al. (2001).

Patient evaluation	Day 1	Day 2	Day 3	Day 4	Day 5
Altered level of consciousness* (A–E)					
If A or B do not complete patient evaluation for the period					
Inattention					
Disorientation					
Hallucination–delusion–psychosis					
Psychomotor agitation or retardation					
Inappropriate speech or mood					
Sleep/wake cycle disturbance					
Symptom fluctuation					
Total score (0–8)					

* Level of consciousness:
A: No response, score: None
B: Response to intense and repeated stimulation (loud voice and pain), score: None
C: Response to mild or moderate stimulation, score: 1
D: Normal wakefulness, score: 0
E: Exaggerated response to normal stimulation, score: 1

Figure 7.2 ▥ Intensive Care Delirium Screening Checklist.
From Bergeron, Dubois, Dumont, Dial, and Skrobik (2001).

Delirium Risk Factors

- Preexisting dementia
- History of baseline hypertension
- Alcoholism
- High severity of illness on admission
- Coma (an independent risk factor)
- Benzodiazepine use

From Barr et al. (2013).

Key Features of Delirium

- A disturbed level of consciousness
- A disturbed clarity of awareness of the environment
- Reduced ability to focus
- Inability to sustain focus or shift focus
- Change in cognition (e.g., memory deficit, disorientation, language disturbance)
- Hallucinations or delusions
- Sleep disturbances
- Emotional disturbances (e.g., fear, anxiety, anger, depression, euphoria, apathy)
- Patients may present as agitated (hyperactive delirium) or calm and lethargic (hypoactive delirium)

NEUROMUSCULAR BLOCKING AGENTS

There has been a substantial decrease in the use of neuromuscular blocking agents (NMBA) in the ICU in recent years (MacIntyre & Branson, 2009). Typically, these agents are used as a last resort when all other modalities have been exhausted. As a first-line approach, every effort should be made to use appropriate sedation and analgesia prior to implementing a neuromuscular blockade regimen for patient/ventilator dysynchrony. Potential indications for neuromuscular blockade include: (a) control of rising intracranial pressure, (b) status epilepticus, (c) induced cooling post–cardiac arrest, and (d) reduced oxygen demands in conditions such as septic shock. Neuromuscular blockade may also be used to facilitate less conventional mechanical ventilation modes such as inverse inspiratory-to-expiratory (I:E) ratios, high-frequency ventilation, and permissive hypercapnia (Pilbeam & Cairo, 2006).

Depolarizing agents (e.g., succinylcholine) are used when short-term blockade is required such as during intubation. These medications bind to and activate nicotinic acetylcholine receptors, which cause initial skeletal muscle stimulation, followed by flaccid muscle paralysis.

Nondepolarizing agents (e.g., pancuronium) bind to acetylcholine receptors but do not cause activation, just paralysis, and are used for longer term blockade.

Nursing management and monitoring of neuromuscular blocking agents includes a number of critical assessments and interventions to ensure patient safety and comfort (see Table 7.4).

Method of Delivery

Neuromuscular blocking agents are initially delivered intravenously with a bolus dose followed by regular doses as necessary (prn) every 1 to 2 hours to maintain blockade. Common nondepolarizing agents include aminosteriods (pancuronium, rocuronium, vecuronium) and benzylisoquinolniums (atracurium, cistracurium, mivacurium). The onset for these drugs ranges from 1 to 4 minutes with a duration of 20 to 116 minutes. Rocuronium has the shortest duration and therefore is a good choice for intubation if other drugs are contraindicated (e.g., succinylcholine). These drugs are typically eliminated via the renal system and cistracurium is a potentially better choice in this category of drugs if there is renal or hepatic failure present; vecuronium is not recommended if liver failure is present.

Table 7.4 ▨ *Caring for a Patient Receiving Neuromuscular Blockade*

Nursing Actions	Rationale
Avoid excessive dosing; titrate drug to individual patient response.	To avoid too much or too little blockade; too much can lead to harmful side effects and prolonged paralysis; too little creates unstable coverage for the patient, which could lead to alterations in hemodynamic stability and patient anxiety
Frequently monitor the IV site.	To ensure delivery of medication and to observe for complications such as thrombophlebitis
Evaluate the depth of blockade by subjective observation and objective grading of muscle activity. One way to analyze muscle activity is through train-of-four twitch monitoring. In this method, two electrodes are placed on the skin along a nerve path near the hand, foot, or facial nerve, then four electrical impulses are delivered to a muscle group in a series and the number of muscle contractions is observed. The degree of blockade is related to the number of contractions elicited (i.e., complete blockade = no contractions, absence of blockade = 4 contractions).	The lowest effective dose should be used
Safety Alert Remember muscles recover in reverse order; therefore, muscular ability of the upper airway is last to return. If the patient cannot hold his or her head off the pillow for longer then 5 seconds then 30% of the receptors are still blocked (Wilson, Collins, & Rowan, 2012).	
Adequate sedation and pain management is essential in patients receiving neuromuscular blockade.	Neuromuscular blocking agents do not provide any sedation or analgesic properties; therefore, it is critical that these drugs be used in combination to provide sedation and comfort to the patient

(continued)

Table 7.4 ▨ (*continued*)

Nursing Actions	Rationale
Ensure patient alarms are on at all times, mechanical ventilation circuit is functioning and intact, and all side rails are in the upright position.	The patient is paralyzed and is not able to call for help if needed
Patients receiving neuromuscular blockade should be cared for in a ratio of 1:1 (nurse: patient) to ensure continuous direct observation.	The patient is paralyzed and is not able to call for help if needed
A sign should be placed above the bed so that other health team members are aware the patient is receiving neuromuscular blockade.	This communicates to other health care team members that the patient is paralyzed
Lubricate eyes with saline drops and cover eyes with saline soaked 2 × 2 gauze.	To prevent corneal abrasions
Frequent patient repositioning (q1–2h); consider use of specialized antipressure beds.	To prevent pressure ulceration
Range-of-motion exercises—passive.	To prevent muscle atrophy and deep vein thrombosis
Keep drug refrigerated.	To promote drug stability
Check incompatibilities carefully prior to administering drug by IV route.	Neuromuscular blocking agents are incompatible with many drugs, including common antibiotics such as cefazolin, ampicillin, and cefotaxime
Auscultate lungs frequently (every 1–2 hours and as necessary) to assess changes in breath sounds; suction by endotracheal tube and orally as needed.	Patient cannot protect the airway; Neuromuscular blockade causes increased salivation
Monitor for abnormal blood gas and electrolyte results.	This can potentiate the action of neuromuscular blockade
Neostigmine is the reversal agent for neuromuscular blockade.	Side effects include bradycardia, bronchospasm, and excessive salivation; in order to minimize these effects, atropine is often administered along with neostigmine

Side effects to monitor for include tachycardia, arrhythmias, hypotension, hypertension, bronchospasm, flushing, and bradycardia.

Complications of Neuromuscular Blockade

Sequelae to neuromuscular blockade are residual neuromuscular blockade, which can contribute to a longer stay in the ICU, are and longer hours of mechanical ventilation. Residual neuromuscular blockade is linked to aspiration, decreased response to hypoxia, and obstruction of the upper airway soon after extubation (Wilson et al., 2012). There are a number of factors that can increase the risk of residual neuromuscular blockade that the critical care nurse should monitor for (see three boxes below).

In order to promote safety in the patient receiving neuromuscular blockade, a clear handoff report is required by the critical care nurse.

Residual Neuromuscular Blockade: Risk Factors

- Renal impairment
- Furosemide, calcium channel blockers, and certain antibiotics (i.e., tobramycin, gentamycin, and clindamycin) have an additive effect
- Hypokalemia, hyponatremia, hypocalcemia, increased magnesium levels, and hypothermia can increase the duration of neuromuscular blockade and extend recovery time.
- Neuromuscular disease (e.g., cerebrovascular accident, Parkinson's, multiple sclerosis, amyotrophic lateral sclerosis (ALS) or myasthenia gravis) can influence neuromuscular blockade.

From Wilson et al. (2012).

Neuromuscular Blockade: Antagonists

- Phenytoin
- Corticosteroids
- Ranitidine

From Baird and Bethel (2011).

Safety Considerations: Analgesia, Sedation, Neuromuscular Blockade

1. Have antidotes available
   - Naloxone for opiates
   - Flumazenil for benzodiazepines
   - Neostigmine and atropine for neuromuscular blockades
2. Have airway equipment available
3. Position patient for full lung expansion
4. Ensure alarms are on at all times
5. Monitor respiratory function and oxygenation closely

ADDITIONAL RESPIRATORY MEDICATIONS IN THE ICU

In addition to the pharmacologic interventions needed for pain, agitation, and sedation, there are other categories of medications the critical care nurse needs to know to provide high-quality care to the patient receiving mechanical ventilation.

Mucolytics

The patient receiving mechanical ventilation can develop excessive pulmonary secretions and mucous plugs that can destabilize the ability to effectively oxygenate the patient. Humidification in the ventilator circuit and patient hydration are important aspects to monitor to prevent secretions from becoming viscous and difficult to remove. It is important to note that adding normal saline to the endotracheal tube is not supported by evidence-based research and may actually be harmful (Seckel, 2012). In some instances, mucolytics such as N-acetylcysteine may be administered; however, there is little evidence to support its use (Ruickbie, Hall, & Ball, 2011).

Bronchodilators

Bronchodilators decrease airway resistance and shortness of breath by relaxing the smooth muscles of the airways. There are three main categories of bronchodilators: beta agonists that stimulate the sympathetic nervous system (e.g., albuterol, salmeterol), anticholinergic agents that block the action of acetylcholine (e.g., atropine, ipratropium), and methylxanthines (e.g., theophylline derivatives) (Pierce, 2007). See Table 7.5 for a description of bronchodilators used in critical care.

Corticosteroids

Corticosteroids are not indicated for rapid response but rather work over hours to days. Corticosteroids can be administered orally, intravenously, or as an aerosol. The action of these medications is as an anti-inflammatory and they operationalize by preventing histamine release, decreasing hypersensitivity reactions, causing edema, and excessive mucous production. Corticosteroids do, however, have a number of local side effects such as fungal infection of the oropharynx, cough bronchospasm, and dysphonia. In addition, the critical care nurse must monitor for such systemic effects as hyperglycemia, fluid retention, sodium retention, potassium loss, gastrointestinal distress and peptic ulcers, steroid psychosis, and impaired healing (Pierce, 2007).

Table 7.5 ▧ *Respiratory Medications*

Bronchodilator	Onset and Duration	Side Effects
Ventolin (albuterol sulfate) Proventil	• Short acting • Onset within minutes • Duration 4 to 6 hours	• Tachycardia • Headache • Tremors • Palpitations
Atrovent (ipratropium bromide)	• Short acting • 5 to 15 minutes • Duration 3 to 6 hours	• Bronchospasm
Atropine	• Short acting • Onset 15 to 30 minutes • Duration 6 to 8 hours	• Tachycardia • Dry mouth • Dilated pupils
Salmeterol	• Long acting • Onset 20 minutes • Duration 12 hours	• Same as above
Spiriva	• Long acting • Duration 24 hours	• Tachycardia • Dry mouth • Urinary retention
Combivent (combination of albuterol and ipratropium)	• See albuterol and ipratropium	

Heliox

Heliox is a mixture of helium and oxygen and is used to decrease the work of breathing in patients with increased airway resistance. Helium augments the effect of CO_2 elimination and improves ventilation perfusion matching through improved alveolar ventilation. The effort needed to move a volume of gas is decreased by one third when breathing helium versus nitrogen (Pierce, 2007). There are no known complications to heliox administration; however, it is an expensive treatment, is temporary, and must be delivered continuously.

Nitric Oxide

Nitric oxide reduces pulmonary resistance by redistributing pulmonary blood flow and decreasing right ventricular work. Nitric oxide enters the blood quickly and combines with hemoglobin, forming methhemoglobin, which serves as a potent pulmonary vasodilator that results in better ventilation perfusion matching and decreased pulmonary vascular resistance. This inhaled agent is used in hypoxic respiratory failure and pulmonary hypertension. Although there are no systemic side effects, nitric oxide must be titrated off gradually because abrupt discontinuation can result in a worsening of the PaO_2 and increase pulmonary artery hypertension. Furthermore, nitric oxide has immunosuppressant properties and can inhibit platelet function (Pierce, 2007).

SUMMARY

In this chapter, current evidence-based guidelines were discussed in relation to pain, agitation, and delirium, along with relevant nursing implications. In addition, other important intensive respiratory care pharmacological treatments for the patient receiving mechanical ventilation were explored in relation to neuromuscular blockade, mucolytics, bronchodilators, corticosteroids, and antipulmonary hypertension agents.

Important Points to Remember

- Analgesia first sedation is to be used in mechanically ventilated ICU patients.
- Improved pain management leads to improved clinical outcomes, such as decreased duration of mechanical ventilation and decreased length of stay in the ICU.

(continued)

Important Points to Remember (*continued*)

- Consider nonpharmacological treatment of pain (e.g., music therapy).
- It is essential to frequently monitor and reassess pain levels.
- ICU patients experience pain even with routine care such as suctioning and repositioning.
- There are short- and long-term consequences to uncontrolled pain (e.g., PTSD).
- Remember to administer pre-emptive analgesia prior to painful procedures.
- Promote sleep by optimizing the patient's environment (e.g., clustering care, decreasing noise and light).
- Daily sedation interruption or a light target level of sedation are recommended in mechanically ventilated patients.
- An interdisciplinary ICU team approach is recommended to facilitate the pain, analgesia, and delirium guidelines that include provider education and protocols.

Adapted from Barr et al. (2013).

Questions to Consider

The answers are found beginning on page 133.

1. Consequences of unrelieved pain in ICU patients can include the following:
   a. Hyperglycemia
   b. Increased risk of infection
   c. PTSD
   d. Sleep disturbances
   e. All of the above
2. Benzodiazepine sedation is associated with increased ICU length of stay. (True or False)
3. The most reliable and valid scale for measuring level of sedation is:
   a. CPOT
   b. BPS
   c. RASS
   d. CAM-ICU
4. What are the risk factors for developing delirium in the ICU?

REFERENCES

AACN (2012). Delirium assessment and management. *Critical Care Nurse, 32*(1), 79–82.

Baird, M., & Bethel, S. (2011). *Manual of critical care nursing.* St. Louis, MO: Elsevier.

Barr, J., Graser, G., Puntillo, K., Ely, E., Gelinas, C., Dasta, J., . . . Jaeske, R. (2013) Clinical practice guidelines for the management of pain, agitation and delirium in adult patients in the intensive care unit. *Critical Care Medicine, 41*(1), 263–306.

Bergeron, N., Dubois, M. J., Dumont, M., Dial, S., & Skrobik, Y. (2001). Intensive care delirium screening checklist: Evaluation of a new screening tool. *Intensive Care Medicine, 27.*

Concepcion, S. (2013). ABCDEs of ICU: Awakening. *Critical Care Nurse Quarterly, 36*(2), 152–156.

Ely, E. W., Inouye, S. K., Bernard, G. R., Gordon, S., Francis, J., May, L., . . . Dittus, R. (2001). Delirium in mechanically ventilated patients: Validity and reliability of the confusion assessment method for the intensive care unit (CAM-ICU). *Journal of the American Medical Association, 286*(21), 2703–2710.

Fraser, G. L., & Riker, R. R. (2001). Monitoring sedation, agitation analgesia, and delirium in critically ill adult patients. *Critical Care Clinics, 17* (4).

Gelinas, C., Fillion, L., & Puntillo, K. (2006). Validation of the critical-care pain observation tool in adult patients. *American Journal of Critical Care, 15*, 420–427.

Karch, A. (2013). *Nursing 2013 drug handbook.* Philadelphia, PA: Lippincott Williams and Wilkins.

MacIntyre, N., & Branson, R. (2009). *Mechanical ventilation* (2nd ed.). St. Louis, MO: Saunders.

Pierce, L. (2007). *Management of the mechanically ventilated patient* (2nd ed.). St. Louis, MO: Elsevier.

Pilbeam, S., & Cairo, J. (2006). *Mechanical ventilation: Physiological and clinical applications* (4th ed.). St. Louis, MO: Elsevier.

Riker, R., Picard, J., & Fraser, G. (1999). Prospective evaluation of the Sedation-Agitation Scale for adult critically ill patients. *Critical Care Medicine*, 27, 1325.

Ruickbie, S., Hall, A., & Ball, J. (2011). Therapeutic aerosols in mechanically ventilated patients. In J. Vincent (Ed.), *Annual update in emergency and critical care medicine* (pp. 197–208). Berlin, Germany: Springer-Verlag.

Seckel, M. (2012). Normal saline and mucous plugging. *Critical Care Nurse, 32*(5), 66–68.

Wilson, J., Collins, A., & Rowan, B. (2012). Residual neuromuscular blockade in critical care. *Critical Care Nurse, 32*(3), e1–e10.

8

International Perspectives and Future Considerations

In this chapter, mechanical ventilation is explored from an international perspective. Future considerations for mechanical ventilation practice are also discussed. Having an understanding about best practices globally can help to inform nurses working in critical care units with critically ill patients who receive mechanical ventilation. Discussions with our international colleagues made it readily apparent that the educational preparation of critical care nurses is quite varied among countries in terms of the availability, accessibility, and level of preparation of nurses who care for patients receiving mechanical ventilation.

INTERNATIONAL PERSPECTIVES

A growing trend in developing countries is the educational strategy of incorporating *high-fidelity simulation* with integrated case-based scenarios to prepare nurses to care for mechanically ventilated patients. These simulated scenarios provide an opportunity for skilled application, development of clinical reasoning, and clinical self-efficacy (Goldsworthy & Graham, 2013). Novice nurses in critical care require additional education beyond basic preparation to enable them to safely and competently care for critically ill patients receiving mechanical ventilation. In the United Kingdom, simulation is used to enhance development of critical care competencies. Students work through full-day scenarios with cases such as a shock scenario to ensure the novice practitioner has the necessary knowledge and skills to manage a critically ill patient.

In Canada, there is a wide variety of educational preparation for critical care nurses. In some regions, the local hospital creates a short course based on the unique needs of the specific patient population. Other courses offered through accredited educational institutions, such as colleges, vary from 3 months to 1 year utilizing both face-to-face and online delivery models. Many critical care courses integrate simulation within their curricula and use this technology to teach complex topics, such as mechanical ventilation, through case-based formats.

To acknowledge the advanced preparation required of a critical care nurse, several countries have a national certification process. Eligibility for the exam is often based on the number of hours worked in critical care, as well as completion of an educational program. Once the critical care nurse has met the competencies for initial certification, ongoing education is required to maintain the certification. To remain current with the national credentialing process, several countries have mandated continuing-education requirements. Attending national critical care conferences or participating in sessions, such as advanced cardiac life support contribute to maintaining ongoing critical care certification.

Globally the composition of health care teams providing care to mechanically ventilated patients varies. Definition of critical care and admission criteria to specialty units is also individual. In some units the nurse patient ratio is 1:1, although in other critical care units the ratio can be 1:2 or 1:3 (Rose, Blackwood, Burns, Frazier, & Egerod, 2012). In the United Kingdom, South Africa, and Canada, the critically ill are managed with a 1:1 ratio, and as the patient stabilizes that ratio may change to 1:2. Teams may vary from country to country; for instance, registered respiratory care practitioners (RRCPs) are, for the most part, unique to North American health care teams. In countries that do not have this category of health professional, mechanical ventilation is primarily managed by the physicians and the critical care nurses.

Management of the patient in the critical care unit continues to challenge health care systems. As a measure to improve patient outcomes and provide cost-effective care, many countries acknowledge the role of the advanced practice nurse. This role is loosely defined depending on the geographic location and the specific needs of the patient population. Each jurisdiction dictates the educational preparation, scope of practice, and credentialing required to fully implement this role in critical care. The advanced practice nurse's role has come under opposition in some countries as physicians see it as an encroachment on their responsibilities. In other countries, despite advanced preparation, this role remains largely restricted (Papathanassoglou, 2011). In countries such as the United States and Canada, the advanced practice role continues to expand and flourish, yet in other countries the advanced practice role remains in the formative stages.

To provide holistic and comprehensive nursing care in the critical care unit to ensure positive patient outcomes, the role of the advanced practice nurse needs to be further refined. This opportunity allows advanced practice nurses to work in the full scope of their practice. Through additional educational preparation at an advanced level, clearly defined regulations, and self-advocacy, this role can fully evolve (Pulcini, Jelic, Gul, & Yuen, 2010). The advanced practice nurse can collaborate with other members of the critical care team to facilitate implementation of evidence-based protocols. The advanced practice nurse can ensure that weaning protocols are initiated, and that early mobilization and enteral feeding are begun in a timely fashion. The role of the advanced practice nurse also encompasses an educational component for the direct care nurse. Through identifying knowledge deficits, the advanced practice nurse can provide educational sessions and ongoing monitoring to facilitate implementation of evidence-based protocols.

A global phenomenon that is confronting the critical care environment is the reliance on newly graduated registered nurses to supplement the workforce. Faced with a shortage of registered nurses (Baumberger-Henry, 2012), new graduates are often recruited to work in the critical care unit. The novice critical care nurse is challenged with higher acuity patients, shorter lengths of stay, and a more complex environment that includes new technologies. Often equipped with only theoretical knowledge, the new graduate has difficulty linking theory to practice (Baumberger-Henry, 2012). This is reflected as a lack of confidence when performing at the bedside. It takes time for the new graduate to develop technical abilities and the clinical judgment required to provide care for the complex critical care patient. The new graduate often lacks the capacity to prioritize in a rapidly changing environment. This lack of nursing experience becomes apparent when the new graduate overlooks the patient in the bed, merely focusing on the technology and equipment around the bedside (S. Schmollgruber, personal communication, March 18, 2013). Further undermining the new graduate's confidence is the lack of support by senior nurses. This is sometimes perceived as personality conflicts or other behaviors that are deemed unsupportive by the new graduate (Baumberger-Henry, 2012). Acculturation to the profession by the senior nurses is necessary to support the new graduates as they transition to this complex and fast-paced environment. The intention must be to provide a supportive and healthy work environment for new graduates so they can focus on providing safe, quality-driven patient care. Recommendations to stem this exodus of new recruits from the ICU are to provide lengthier orientations and mentoring by the senior nurses. Another strategy to further support the new graduate in developing confidence, clinical judgment, and the reflective practice required in critical care, is the establishment of a 1-year nurse residency program unique to the specific practice environment (Benner, Sutphen, Leonard, Day, & Shulman, 2010). Through supportive mentoring, the new graduate learns to feel comfortable and can contribute positively to this environment.

WHAT DOES THE FUTURE HOLD?

To engage in evidence-based practice, there is a need for further research into standardized evidence-based protocols. Implementation of these standardized protocols, such as prevention of ventilator-acquired pneumonia, has resulted in improved patient outcomes. Nurse scientists need to engage with the direct care nurse to gain an understanding of challenges to implementation of evidence-based practices. This dialogue will also share new protocols and standards with the direct care nurse. Armed with the scientific evidence to support these standardized protocols allows a dialogue beyond nursing with the interprofessional team. Using a team-based approach will foster a collaborative plan of care to promote timely progression of the critically ill patient through the acute illness phase to the rehabilitative phase.

Nursing management of the patient requiring mechanical ventilation requires advanced and sophisticated interventions. Critical care nurses require education and expert mentoring to safely and competently provide the evidence-based care necessary for these patients. Quality research is required to validate the importance of standardized approaches to the mechanically ventilated patient.

> **Clinical Pearl**
>
> To standardize educational practices for the care of patients requiring mechanical ventilation, expand on consortiums (e.g., World Confederation of Critical Care Nurses) to create working groups dedicated to implementing standardized protocols. These groups would have a mandate to include developed and underdeveloped countries in educational initiatives. By supporting nurses in countries in which a patriarchal system of health care may exist, critical care nurses may feel empowered through education, while at the same time be able to bring evidence-based practice to the bedside.

REFERENCES

Baumberger-Henry, M. (2012). Registered nurses' perspectives on the new graduate working in the emergency department or critical care unit. *The Journal of Continuing Education in Nursing, 43*(7), 299–305. doi: 10.3928/00220124-2011115-02

Benner, P., Sutphen, M., Leonard, V., Day, L., & Shulman, L. (2010). *A call for radical transformation.* San Fransisco, CA: Jossey-Bass.

Goldsworthy, S., & Graham, L. (2013). *Simulation simplified: A practical guide for nurse educators.* Philadelphia, PA: Lippincott Williams and Wilkins.

Papathanassoglou, E. (2011). Advanced critical care nursting: A novel role with ancient history and unprecedented challenges worldwide. *British Association of Critical Care Nurses, 16*(2), 55–57.

Pulcini, J., Jelic, M., Gul, R., & Yuen, A. (2010). An international survey on advanced practice education, practice and regulation. *Journal of Nursing Scholarship, 42*(1), 31–39. doi: 10.1111/j.1547-5069.2009.01322

Rose, L., Blackwood, B., Burns, S., Frazier, S., & Egerod, I. (2011). International perspectives on the influence of structure and process of weaning from mechanical ventilation. *American Journal of Critical Care, 20*, e10–e18. doi: 10.4037/ajcc2011430

Answers to "Questions to Consider"

CHAPTER 1

1.

Pulmonary embolism	Dead-space unit
Atelectasis	Shunt unit
Cardiac arrest	Silent unit

2. Decreased cardiac output, fever, pain, decreased hemoglobin, and anxiety can cause decreased oxygen delivery to cells and influence SVO_2 levels.

3. Early signs of oxygen toxicity include, substernal chest pain, dry cough, dyspnea, restlessness, and lethargy.

CHAPTER 2

1.
- Acute respiratory failure
- Unable to stabilize the chest wall (e.g., trauma, flail chest, penetrating injuries)
- After major surgery to maintain oxygenation
- Cardiogenic or septic shock to decrease myocardial workload and maintain oxygenation
- Severe asthma
- ARDS (acute respiratory distress syndrome)
- Pneumonia
- Burns and smoke inhalation
- Neuromuscular disease (e.g., Guillian–Barré, ALS, myasthenia gravis)
- Overdose
- Brainstem injury
- COPD (e.g., emphysema, cystic fibrosis)

2. • Vital capacity < 10 mL/kg
   • Unable to achieve maximal inspiratory force to −25 cm H_2O
   • PaO_2 < 60 mmHg with an FiO_2 of > .50 (oxygenation issue)
   • pH < 7.25 (ventilation issue)
   • Arterial PaO_2 < 30 or > 50
   • Dead space /tidal volume ratio 0.6
   • Respiratory rate > 35/min

3.

ARDS Severity	PaO_2/FiO_2 ratio
Mild	200–300
(previously called acute lung injury [ALI])	
Moderate	100–200
Severe	< 100

4. a.
5. b.

Case Study

1. Common triggers of asthma are: a respiratory infection, allergens, smoke, and extreme anxiety.
2. Bronchospasm, further hypoxemia
3. Hydration, psychosocial support, treatment of infection as appropriate, and close monitoring of changes in respiratory status and vital signs.

CHAPTER 3

1.

Pressure-Targeted Ventilation	Volume-Targeted Ventilation
• The ventilator delivers the breath until the preset inspiratory pressure has been reached	• Each breath delivered by the ventilator has the same tidal volume
• The patient receives variable tidal volumes depending on lung compliance and airway resistance	• The ventilator rate is set
	• The volume is delivered and is not dependent on lung compliance or resistance

(continued)

Pressure-Targeted Ventilation	Volume-Targeted Ventilation
	• The patient will receive a predetermined minute volume • If the peak inspiratory pressure reaches the alarm limit that has been set, the remainder of the tidal volume will be terminated

2. Assist/control ventilation can be used for a patient emerging from anesthesia as the patient has a normal respiratory drive but the respiratory muscles are weak.

3. Measures to optimize the ventilator settings to decrease the work of breathing, such as titrating sensitivity or peak inspiratory flow to meet the patient's needs. It may be necessary to change to another mode of ventilation. Assess for an increase in airway resistance, rule out causes such herniation of the cuff of the ETT (endotracheal tube), or increased secretions. The use of sedation may be necessary after other causes of dyssynchrony have been ruled out.

Case Study

1. BiPAP noninvasive ventilation
2. Low pressure, high pressure, and apnea
3. The most appropriate mode is pressure-control ventilation. The patient would require an endotracheal tube placed by the designated health care provider; ventilator settings selected and documented by the designated health care provider or the nurse; a respiratory assessment, including auscultating the chest, monitoring vital signs, SaO_2, and hemodynamic status; a chest x-ray, routinely performed to assess endotracheal tube placement; and ABGs (arterial blood gases) 20 minutes after intubation to assess the effectiveness of the intervention.

CHAPTER 4

1. Metabolic acidosis with partial compensation and mild hypoxemia
2. • Establish a communication-friendly environment (e.g., reduce extraneous noise, consider lighting, face the patient at eye level).
   • Assess functional skills related to communication (e.g., does the patient need glasses or a hearing aid?; can he or she hold a pencil?).
   • To reduce anxiety, anticipate the patient's needs.

- Have the clipboard and pencil at the bedside and encourage the patient to write down basic needs.
- Share with the patient's family and other health care team members communication strategies to assist the patient.

3. To assist in preventing ventilator-associated pneumonia (VAP) by decreasing the opportunity for aspiration

4. Causes of high-pressure alarms include:

- Increased pulmonary secretions
- Patient biting ETT
- Ventilator tubing kinked
- ETT cuff herniation
- Increased airway resistance
  (i.e., bronchospasm, coughing, pneumonia, acute respiratory distress syndrome (ARDS), pneumothorax, pulmonary edema, atelectasis, worsening of underlying disease process)
- Patient/ventilator asynchrony
- Water in ventilator circuitry
- Change in position that restricts wall movement

5.
- Minimize noise, especially loud sudden noises during the night.
- Provide access to natural light to avoid the patient losing track of day/night cycles (avoid bright lights and harsh fluorescent lighting wherever possible, especially in the middle of the night).
- Offer relaxation techniques (e.g., progressive muscle relaxation, massage—especially hands, feet, shoulders).
- Communicate with the patient and the patient's family to determine the patient's normal sleep patterns.
- Offer music intervention (consider patient preference, proper volume, and duration).
- Provide animal-assisted therapy (develop a policy on pet visitation).
- Imagery
- Offer presence (physical, psychological, active listening; be attentive to the patient).
- Try to promote periods of uninterrupted sleep by clustering interventions and assessments together; sleep is essential in promoting healing.
- Ensure comfortable positioning, smooth sheets and lift sheets.

6. The patient is becoming septic. Initiate institutional policy for sepsis management: monitor temperature, heart rate, blood pressure, RR, white blood cell. Obtain samples for pan cultures, complete blood count (CBC) with differential, ABGs, lactate, chemistry, clotting studies, chest x-ray, and ECG. Be prepared to initiate fluid resuscitation; administer antibiotics, and stabilize B/P with vasopressors, support oxygenation and ventilation with mechanical ventilation.

7. The large radiolucent area indicates easy penetration of the x-ray to indicate excess air. The absence of vascular markings, a new lung margin that is not in contact with the chest wall, as well as deviation of the trachea indicates a tension pneumothorax. This is an emergency situation requiring needle decompression.

Case Study

1. Connect to monitoring devices and assess pulse oximetry and end tidal CO_2; provide telemetry for arrhythmias, zero arterial lines; assess vital signs including pain level.
2. Complete a head-to-toe assessment with a focused cardiorespiratory assessment. Assess for a mediastinal shift toward the operative side as the good lung can encroach the vacant lung field. Assess for postoperative hemorrhage.
3. Regulate intravenous therapy to minimum required to prevent post-pneumonectomy fluid overload and subsequent pulmonary edema.
4. Position patient supine or on operative side to splint the incision and facilitate deep breathing.
5. Initiate postoperative orders for ECG, chest x-ray, and baseline blood samples for CBC, chemistry, arterial blood gases, cardiac markers, liver function tests, glucose, renal function, and coagulation profiles.

CHAPTER 5

1.

Short-Term Ventilation	Long-Term Ventilation
• Less than 3 days • Often used for elective procedures, respiratory distress related to disease processes such as congestive heart failure or trauma	• Greater than 3 days • Used for patients who failed short-term weaning • Patients often have multiple comorbidities

(continued)

Short-Term Ventilation	Long-Term Ventilation
• Often extubated quickly	• Often requires a tracheostomy to facilitate weaning • May take days to weeks to wean from ventilator

2.

Weaning Technique	Advantage
Pressure support	Provides inspiratory support to overcome the resistance of the ETT; decreases the work of breathing
T-piece	Patient performs all of the work of breathing without support of the ventilator
CPAP	Augments oxygenation, allows patient to perform work of breathing
SIMV	Very gradual decrease in ventilator support

3. Patient is stable and prepared for extubation. Suctioned for a scant amount of mucoid secretions via ETT and orally. Patient extubated and placed on FiO_2 0.40 per face mask. Chest expansion symmetrical, air entry bilateral with decreased breath sounds throughout. Vital signs stable, SaO_2 95%. Patient remains in sinus rhythm, no ectopy noted. Postextubation ABGs obtained.

Case Study

1. Assessment:
   - Complete a weaning tool, such as the Burns Wean Assessment Program
   - Assess chest x-ray for improvement
   - Monitor vital signs, cardiac monitor for stability
   - Assess patient's anxiety and readiness to wean
   - Obtain ABGs, end tidal carbon dioxide, and oxygen saturation
2. To facilitate successful weaning:
   - Long periods of rest
   - Adequate nutritional status

- Interprofessional collaboration
- Early tracheotomy
3. To extubate Mr. Snider:
  - Assess respiratory status
  - Ensure qualified personnel is available for potential reintubation
  - Discontinue feeding tubes 4 to 6 prior to extubation
  - Hyperoxygenate and suction ETT and the pharynx
  - Remove securement device or tapes
  - Deflate cuff and instruct the patient to take a deep breath
  - Remove the ETT at peak inspiration
  - Encourage patient to deep breathe and cough
  - Apply supplemental oxygen
  - Monitor respiratory status, oxygen saturation, vital signs, presence of stridor or hoarseness, presence of larngospasm, arterial blood gases
  - Be prepared to institute invasive or noninvasive ventilation

CHAPTER 6

1. • Discharge to a step-down unit or progressive care unit
   - Discharge to an inpatient respiratory unit
   - Discharge to a long-term care unit
   - Discharge to a rehabilitation unit
   - Discharge home
2. • Discuss with the patient her or his wishes for discharge
   - Identify and invite the team
   - Plan a weaning schedule, including milestones
3. • Notify the receiving unit of arrival time
   - Have respiratory therapist accompany patient and nurse on transfer
   - Ensure family is aware of transfer
   - Secure all lines
   - Fully engage the monitoring system: cardiac monitor, B/P, pulse oximetry, ventilator alarms
   - Have the respiratory therapist at the head of the bed to observe the patient's airway; position the nurse at the foot of the bed to observe the monitor and the patient's overall appearance
   - Have emergency equipment available

Case Study

1. Key priorities:
   - Perform respiratory assessment and ausculate chest
   - Perform ventilator assessment
   - Request that the respiratory therapist assess patient
   - Place patient in high Fowler's position
   - Provide reassurance to make the patient feel safe in the new environment
   - Pharmacological intervention as ordered
2. Advocacy includes:
   - Discuss wishes for discharge with Mrs. Mills
   - Identify and invite the interprofessional team to a team conference
   - Plan collaborative care based on standardized protocols and evidence based practice

CHAPTER 7

1. e.
2. True.
3. c.
4.
   - Preexisting dementia
   - History of baseline hypertension
   - Alcoholism
   - High severity of illness on admission
   - Coma (an independent risk factor)
   - Benzodiazepine use

Glossary

Absorptive atelectasis In this situation, high concentrations of O_2 wash out the nitrogen that usually holds the alveoli open at the end of expiration.

Acinus Refers to the terminal respiratory unit distal to the terminal bronchioles, which uses an alveolar membrane for gas exchange.

Alveolar ventilation Refers to the volume of air per minute that participates in gas exchange.

Anatomic dead space Refers to the volume of air in conducting airways that does not participate in gas exchange.

Arterial blood gas (ABG) An arterial blood sample provides information about the patient's oxygenation, ventilation, and acid–base status.

Arterial chemoreceptors Found within the aortic arch and carotid bodies; sensitive to levels of pH and PaO_2.

Atelectrauma Ventilator-induced lung injury related to unstable alveoli repeatedly opening and closing.

Baroreceptors Found in the aortic arch and carotid bodies; they can increase blood pressure in response to cardiac output changes, which in turn can inhibit ventilation.

Barotrauma Occurs when an overdistended alveolus ruptures or is injured.

Central chemoreceptors Sensitive to cerebral spinal fluid pH, they are the primary control of ventilation, and are influenced by levels of $PaCO_2$ and pH.

Compliance The measurement of extensibility of lung tissue.

Dead-space ventilation Refers to the volume of air per minute that does not participate in gas exchange.

High-fidelity simulation The use of a programmable manikin that replicates human heart sounds, breathing sounds, bowel sounds, and other characteristics to mimic a real patient.

Hypoxemic pulmonary vasoconstriction Can occur in a localized or generalized manner when oxygen flow is decreased to the lungs.

Minute ventilation The volume of air inhaled and exhaled per minute.

Negative inspiratory pressure A measurement performed when the patient is connected to a series of one-way valves and a manometer in which the patient inspires against a closed system to determine the strength of the inspiratory muscles.

Orthopnea Refers to shortness of breath when the patient is in a recumbent position.

Oxygen toxicity Occurs in patients breathing a concentration of oxygen greater than 50% longer than 24 hours; signs and symptoms of oxygen toxicity include pulmonary edema and acute lung injury if high oxygen levels are delivered for a prolonged period.

Paradoxical breathing Abnormal breathing pattern in which the chest rises on inspiration and the abdomen is drawn in or flattened due to respiratory muscle fatigue.

Paroxysmal nocturnal dyspnea Sudden onset of respiratory distress during sleep.

Peak inspiratory pressure The highest pressure in the lung during a ventilator breath.

Positive end expiratory pressure (PEEP) Pressure exerted by the ventilator at the end of expiration that increases the volume and pressure within the alveoli resulting in improved oxygenation. Common levels are 5 to 15 cm. May be dialed in by the ventilator or spontaneously by the patient known as auto-PEEP; auto-PEEP is caused by obstruction to airflow.

Prolonged mechanical ventilation Refers to a patient requiring a mechanical ventilator for longer than 21 days.

Proprioreceptors Located in the muscles and tendons and increase ventilation in response to body movement.

Rapid shallow breathing index A test calculated by dividing the respiratory rate or frequency by the tidal volume (i.e., f/V_T) to determine weaning status (normal is 60–105; less than 105 indicates that weaning is more likely to successful; greater than 105 indicates the patient is not ready for the weaning trial).

Resistance The measurement of the forces impeding air flow.

Spontaneous breathing trial Assessment done prior to discontinuation of the mechanical ventilator the during which patient breathes spontaneously on a low level of constant positive airway pressure (CPAP), such as 5 cm, or has low-level pressure support, such as 5 to 8 cm, or on a T-piece for 30 to 120 minutes.

Tidal volume The volume of air inhaled and exhaled with each breath.

Vital capacity The maximum volume of air exhaled from the point of maximal inspiration.

Volutrauma Refers to excessive alveolar stretch caused by end-inspiratory overdistension, which results in stress on alveolar–capillary membrane, which leads to increased permeability of the alveolar–capillary membrane and pulmonary edema.

Index